The Complete Guide to Core Surgical Training Interviews

The Complete Guide to Core Surgical Training Interviews

Oliver Skan
Core Surgical Trainee, London

Kiran Saini
Core Surgical Trainee, Oxford

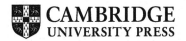

CAMBRIDGE
UNIVERSITY PRESS

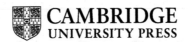

CAMBRIDGE
UNIVERSITY PRESS

Shaftesbury Road, Cambridge CB2 8EA, United Kingdom

One Liberty Plaza, 20th Floor, New York, NY 10006, USA

477 Williamstown Road, Port Melbourne, VIC 3207, Australia

314–321, 3rd Floor, Plot 3, Splendor Forum, Jasola District Centre,
New Delhi – 110025, India

103 Penang Road, #05–06/07, Visioncrest Commercial, Singapore 238467

Cambridge University Press is part of Cambridge University Press &
Assessment, a department of the University of Cambridge.

We share the University's mission to contribute to society through the
pursuit of education, learning and research at the highest international
levels of excellence.

www.cambridge.org
Information on this title: www.cambridge.org/9781009520102

DOI: 10.1017/9781009520096

First published 2025

A catalogue record for this publication is available from the British Library.

*A Cataloging-in-Publication data record for this book is available from the
Library of Congress*

ISBN 978-1-009-52010-2 Paperback

Cambridge University Press & Assessment has no responsibility for the
persistence or accuracy of URLs for external or third-party internet websites
referred to in this publication and does not guarantee that any content on
such websites is, or will remain, accurate or appropriate.

. . . .

Contents

Preface

Welcome to *The Complete Guide to Core Surgical Training Interviews*. We applied for CST in 2022–2023 and recall how daunting and opaque the process can feel. It is a competitive and time-consuming application process that for many is completed while also working busy jobs in the NHS.

Like many candidates, we identified that the interview, heavily weighted as it is, is where you can best earn yourself a high ranking. We produced our own approaches to the clinical, ethical, and leadership stations, which we practised together repeatedly in the run-up to the interview. While revising, we felt that no individual textbook or online revision resource covered the interview in the depth and breadth we felt was necessary to ensure a candidate can stand out in what is a highly competitive field.

We were very fortunate to rank first and second nationally in 2023 and were able to obtain our top-choice jobs. We decided to put our methods down on paper and try to create a definitive text on the interview process. We hope it might be of some use to you.

Acknowledgements

We would like to thank the following colleagues and mentors for lending their assistance and expertise to help make this book possible by serving as expert reviewers for the different specialties:

Dr Sarah Al-Rawi MBBS, MmedSc, MRCPCH

    Specialty Registrar – Paediatrics
    Northwick Park Hospital

Miss Ann Agayby MBBCh, MRCS

    Core Surgical Trainee (CT2) – General Surgery
    Oxford University Hospitals NHS Foundation Trust

Mr Usama Ahmed MRCS, DOHNS

    Specialty Registrar – Otolaryngology and Head & Neck Surgery
    Northwick Park Hospital

Miss Camille Anne Aliker BMBS, BMedSci(Hons), MRCS

    Specialty Registrar – Trauma and Orthopaedic Surgery
    Royal Free London NHS Foundation Trust

Mr Orestis Argyriou MSc, MRCSEd

    Research Fellow in IBD & Colorectal Surgery
    Specialty Registrar – General Surgery
    St Mark's National Bowel Hospital and Academic Institute

Mr Soham Bandyopadhyay MA, BMBCh(Oxon), PGCert, AFHEA, MPHMRCS, AdvDip, HFMA, FioL, FRSPH, FRSA

    Academic Clinical Fellow (ST2) – Neurosurgery
    University of Southampton

Mr David Drake

    Retired Pediatric Surgeon and Volunteer Lecturer
    King's College London

Dr Elif Iliria Emin MBBS, BSc, PGCert (Clinical Ed)

    Specialty Registrar (ST1) – Obstetrics & Gynaecology
    North Central East London Deanery

Mr Michael Fadel BSc(Hons), MBBS, MRCS

    NIHR Doctoral Fellow & Specialty Registrar – General Surgery
    Department of Surgery and Cancer, Imperial College London

Mr Naim Fakih-Gomez

Consultant – Bariatric & UGI Surgery
Chelsea and Westminster NHS Foundation Trust

Mr Matthew Harris MBBS, FRCS

Specialty Registrar – Vascular Surgery
Royal Free Hospital

Miss Belinda Hughes MBChB, MRCS

Specialty Registrar – General Surgery
St Thomas' Hospital

Miss Nikita Joji MBChB, BSc(Hons), MRCS(Eng), MSc(MedEd)

Specialty Registrar – Plastic Surgery
Royal Free Hospital

Dr Aaron Leiblich FRCS (Urol), Dphil

Consultant – Urology
Oxford University Hospitals NHS Foundation Trust

Mr Vinay Shah BSc(Hons), MBBS (Dist.), AICSM, MRCS(Eng), PGCert(MedEd)

Specialty Registrar – Trauma and Orthopaedic Surgery

Dr Michail Sideris MD, MDRes, PhD, MRCOG

Subspecialty Trainee – Gynaecological Oncology
The Royal London Hospital

Dr JN Spence MBChB (Hons), BSc (Hons)

Surgical Physician
John Radcliffe Hospital

Mr Sebastian Vaughan-Burleigh BMBCh(Oxon), MA(Hons), MRCS

Academic Clinical Fellow – Vascular Surgery
Oxford University Hospitals

Dr Jessica Whitburn MBBS, PGDip, DPhil, FRCS(Urol.)

Specialty Registrar – Urology
Oxford University Hospitals NHS Foundation Trust

Mr Gentle Wong FRCS(ORL-HNS)

Consultant – Otolaryngology
Northwick Park Hospital

We also thank the following colleagues for their advice and help, or for contributing example speeches to the text:

Dr Edward Armstrong BA(Oxon), MBBS

Core Surgical Trainee (CT1)
Oxford University Hospitals NHS Foundation Trust

Dr Burhan Mirza MBBS, MRes, BSc(Hons)

Core Surgical Trainee (CT1) – Trauma & Orthopaedics
Wexham Park Hospital

Mr Nithesh Ranasinha BMBCh, BA(Hons), MRCS, PGCert(MedEd)

Core Surgical Trainee (CT1)
Oxford University Hospitals NHS Foundation Trust

Mr Iolo Thomas-Jones BSc (Hons), MB ChB, PGCert (Clin.Ed.)

Core Surgical Trainee (CT1) – Trauma & Orthopaedics
Maidstone and Tunbridge Wells Hospital

Abbreviations

ABG	arterial blood gas
Abx	antibiotics
ACF	antecubital fossa
AKI	acute kidney injury
ARDS	acute respiratory distress syndrome
AVPU	Alert, Voice, Pain, Unresponsive
AXR	abdominal X-ray
BP	blood pressure
CAP	community-acquired pneumonia
COPD	chronic obstructive pulmonary disease
CRP	c-reactive protein
CRT	capillary refill time
CTG	cardiotocography
CXR	chest X-ray
DGH	district general hospital
EDL	extensor digitorum longus
EGFR	estimated glomerular filtration rate
EHL	extensor hallucis longus
EWTD	European working time directive
FAST	focused assessment with sonography in trauma
FDL	flexor digitorum longus
FFP	fresh frozen plasma
FNA	fine needle aspirate
GCS	Glasgow coma scale
HAP	hospital-acquired pneumonia
HCG	human chorionic gonadotrophin
HR	heart rate
LDH	lactate dehydrogenase
LFT	liver function tests
LUTS	lower urinary tract symptoms
MDT	multidisciplinary team
NBM	nil by mouth
NGT	nasogastric tube
NOK	next of kin
OGD	oesophagogastroduodenoscopy
OSA	obstructive sleep apnoea
PCC	prothrombin complex concentrate
PE	pulmonary embolism
PR	per rectum
RA	room air
RBC	red blood cells
RR	respiratory rate
SBAR	Situation, Background, Assessment, Recommendation
U&Es	urea and electrolytes
UGIB	upper gastrointestinal bleeding
UO	urine output
VBG	venous blood gas
VRII	variable rate insulin infusion

Introduction

1.1 Overview of Core Surgical Training Applications

Core surgical training (CST) is a critical step in the journey to becoming a surgeon in the UK. This two-year training programme should equip trainees with the skills required to step up to speciality training. It is a highly selective process which appears to only be getting more competitive. Data from NHS England shows that competition ratios have been increasing steadily for the last decade, from 1.92:1 in 2013 to 4:17 in 2023 (Figure 1.1) [1].

This is because while applicants have effectively doubled in this time (1,296 applicants in 2013 compared to 2,539 applicants in 2023) the number of CST posts has, remarkably, fallen (676 posts in 2013 compared to 609 posts in 2023).

The recent introduction of the MSRA (Multi-Speciality Recruitment Assessment) as part of the application requirements may make the process of getting an interview even more competitive, and it is noteworthy that there was an increase of around 10% in the number of CST applicants in 2023 (the year the MSRA was introduced). Candidates who have been required to sit the MSRA for another specialty are incentivised to also apply for CST – having already done the examination, why not? While a higher volume of applicants will make getting an interview more difficult, this same logic follows that once you have secured an interview the field should be slightly weaker, as it will contain applicants for whom CST is not their first-choice training pathway.

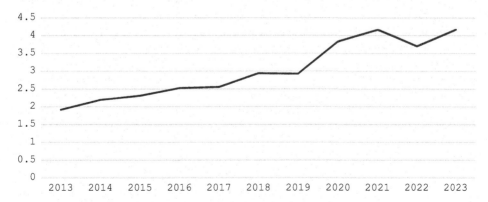

Figure 1.1 Change in competition ratios (y-axis) over time (x-axis) from 2013 to 2023.
Data obtained from NHS England: medical.hee.nhs.uk/medical-training-recruitment/medical-specialty-training/competition-ratios © Crown copyright, reproduced under the Open Government Licence.

Given these competition ratios, getting any CST post is an achievement. Unfortunately, getting specific specialty rotations is particularly important for core surgical trainees as when applicants finish CST and apply for ST3 (the first year of specialty training), core operative procedures form a sizeable chunk of an applicant's portfolio. Different specialties have different procedures that you score on. How difficult these are to achieve vary by specialty; at the time of writing, orthopaedics currently only scores for 'operations for fracture of neck of femur', with top marks available for completing 12 or more of these. By comparison, plastic surgery ST3 applications score on a vast range of burns, skin cancer, and hand trauma procedures, requiring a high level of operative proficiency to score well in. It is highly unlikely you will achieve these requirements without sufficient time in your chosen speciality, which will make applying for ST3 more difficult. More to the point, life as an ST3 will be very difficult if you are not confident in these core procedures. Therefore, getting a CST rank high enough to get any job is laudable, but ideally you want to be able to pick a job that has your chosen specialty as at least one of the rotations (assuming you know what specialty you are keen on pursuing). Of the roughly 600 jobs available, around 400 are 'themed' around a particular specialty, which provide trainees with good exposure to that specialty and the allied specialties related to it. It goes without saying that your CST ranking will also determine where in the country you will be carrying out your training, which for many people is even more important than what rotations they are given.

This is not meant to cause anxiety, but to highlight how essential it is to give your best possible performance in your interview. Of course, there will always be scope to complete clinical fellowships before or after CST to gain the required experience, swapping jobs is possible within some deaneries, and indeed many candidates are not sure what specialty they want to pursue until they have already started CST. Regardless, you should put yourself in a position where you can achieve the highest ranking possible, so that you are the one making the choices about your career.

1.2 How to Use This Book

This book is designed to be read in order, and each chapter is designed with progression in mind. The introduction to the clinical and ethical cases are essential reading, which demonstrate the basic approach we subsequently use for all cases. Cases are initially written out verbatim *in italics* to highlight this structure. However, as a chapter progresses, cases are answered using bullet points to allow candidates to practise generating their own longform answers. At this point, we stop repeating many of the basic points of the approach, which we expect readers to have picked up. It is therefore vital that the introduction and early cases are read, and candidates are confident in this structure, before progressing to the later cases. We revert to verbatim answers intermittently throughout the textbook to remind candidates of the structure and flow of a full model answer.

There is also progression within each case. A strong A–E clinical assessment, or I-SPIES-DR ethical scenario approach is essential in almost all cases. This will take up most of the time in the station and be responsible for most of the marks available. The follow-up questions are there to stretch candidates. In many scenarios it would be impossible in five minutes to complete an A–E assessment as well as answering all of the questions. Some of the follow-up questions are difficult, and may be beyond what is expected at the interview, but have been chosen to highlight clinically important areas and provide a depth of knowledge that would allow you to stand out as an exceptional candidate. You should avoid the temptation of practising in-depth follow-up questions (which may or may not come up) before you can list your basic approach to any scenario confidently and smoothly. The interviewers are looking for prospective surgical trainees who can safely manage patients out of hours, not people who understand the intricacies of a Whipple's procedure!

Please note that we have aimed to ensure all the clinical information provided is uncontroversial and found in reputable sources such as BOASts (British Orthopaedic Association standards for Trauma and Orthopaedics) or NICE guidelines. Moreover, all clinical stations have been checked by specialty doctors. However, this book is not a clinical resource, and you should not be using it to manage patients in your day job. This is a text specifically to help you approach the CST interviews and should not be used to guide the clinical management of patients in real-world settings.

1.3 How to Prepare for the Interview

We recommend preparing for the interview in a small group. Ideally, practise with people who want to put in a similar amount of time over a similar timescale as you, who will push you to improve, and from whom you think you can learn. Identify one or two other candidates to practise with regularly. Regular practice with the same partner will allow you to be more honest with each other about areas that need improvement and allow you to see one another's progression more clearly. Closer to the interview it is helpful to practise with a wider variety of colleagues to help you finesse your technique.

Before you start, make a list of all the possible interview scenarios that you think could reasonably come up (this book will serve as a good guide for this), which you can add to over time as you think of other potential cases. It might feel repetitive, but when going through cases make sure you are doing a full A–E approach (or I-SPIES-DR workup for management cases) each time, making the small changes necessary to fit your template to the scenario at hand. Whilst practising, avoid the temptation to skip straight to the management or follow-up questions – every time you complete your A–E approach you will help embed this to memory, while also picking up small points where you might be able to shave off a few seconds or sound a bit slicker in future cases.

When you practise follow-up questions, get into the habit of structuring your answers. For example, postoperative complications can be listed as 'immediate, early, and late', risk factors as 'modifiable and non-modifiable', aetiology as 'infective, neoplastic, vascular, inflammatory, traumatic etc'. Having a logical structure will give you something to fall back on, buying you time to consolidate your thoughts, while also giving you prompts to jog your memory. You will come across as significantly more confident than if trying to list things off the top of your head.

As you continue to practise, do not stick too rigorously to the listed scenario – you will quickly rote learn this. Instead, vary the scenarios as you go through. For example, interrupt the other person during their A–E by presenting them with an unexpected complication during their resuscitation, vary how acutely unwell the patient is, add an important comorbidity into the stem, or throw in an angry family member to complicate things. While the scenarios given in the book may be similar to what you would expect in an interview, they won't be identical. It's important you develop the ability to think on your feet and are able to change direction in the middle of a scenario if needed. Embedding the fundamentals to memory will free up thinking space for you to adapt during the interview. Similarly with some management scenarios we have given examples of ways the cases could be altered to slightly change the scenario – this will allow you to practise cases in multiple ways.

Reference

1. Health Education England (n.d.). 'Competition ratios'. NHS, Website, accessed 19 Feb. 2024, https://medical.hee.nhs.uk/medical-training-recruitment/medical-specialty-training/competition-ratios.

The MSRA

Chapter 2

2.1 Overview of the MSRA

100% of Shortlisting for Interview & 10% of Overall Score

The Multi-Specialty Recruitment Assessment (MSRA) is a computer-based exam used to test clinical problem-solving skills and professional behaviour. The examination is free and is taken in a two-week window during the application process (January for the 2022/2023 cycle). It is carried out at Pearson Vue centres in the UK.

During the 2022/2023 cycle, this examination was introduced as a new method of shortlisting candidates for interview. It was introduced predominantly to deal with the problem of portfolio verification. Prior to 2022 candidates were shortlisted for interviews based on their portfolio scores. This required examiners to assess each portfolio in turn to verify that the score the candidate had assigned to their portfolio was correct. This labour-intensive process could not keep up with the rise in CST applicants. As justification for introducing the examination, the Joint Committee for Surgical Training (JCST) noted that of those CST applicants who had taken the MSRA over the preceding three years for other training programmes, there was a statistically significant difference in the mean score for those invited to interview compared to those who were not.

There was a strong backlash from several trainee bodies at the time, but it looks like the examination is here to stay, and as such, this general medical examination will determine if you get an interview or not. In 2022–2023, it whittled a field of 2,539 applicants down to just 1,075 candidates invited to interview. Scoring a good mark is vital, else your hard work on your portfolio and interview preparation will be for nothing. A strong showing will also help prop up your overall ranking as this examination contributes 10% to your total score. There will be fantastic surgical candidates who underestimate this exam and find themselves without an interview. Dedicate regular time to this exam for at least three months, take study leave near the exam, and treat this as a priority.

The examination consists of two parts – Professional Dilemmas (PD) and Clinical Problem Solving (CPS). The PD paper consists of 50 questions in 90 minutes and places the candidate in the context of an F2 doctor approaching various workplace scenarios. The candidate must rank the appropriateness of the provided responses between 1 and 5. This is a 'situational judgement test' style approach which tests a candidate's professional integrity, their ability to cope with pressure, and their empathy and sensitivity. The CPS paper involves 97 questions delivered over 75 minutes. The questions are either extended

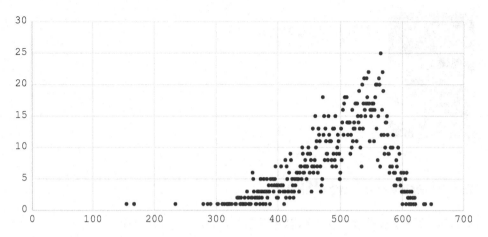

Figure 2.1 Number of candidates (y-axis) achieving a given MSRA score (x-axis) for the 2022–2023 application cycle.
Data obtained via Freedom of Information Act request to Health Education England 24 July 2022, FOI-2307-2006479 NHSE:0176379. © Crown copyright, reproduced under the Open Government Licence.

matching questions or single best answer questions. Note that around 10% of the questions are 'pilot' questions being tested for future examinations, and do not count towards a candidate's final score. This paper tests your broad medical knowledge, and there is minimal surgical knowledge tested in the paper.

2.2 Preparing for the MSRA

We would strongly recommend subscribing to one or more online question banks. Examples of online resources include PassTest, PassMedicine, MediBuddy, eMedica, and MCQBank. Use the resources you feel are most reasonably priced, have the level of depth you desire, and have the interface you prefer. In our experience and through discussion with colleagues, we feel MCQBank is most like the exam and PassMedicine is the easiest format to learn content from, but they all have their advantages and disadvantages. We would recommend using more than one and having completed each question bank more than once.

Nationally, MSRA scores fit a normal distribution around a mean of 500. A freedom of information request obtained the MSRA scores of all candidates for 2022–2023, shown in Figure 2.1.

The average score for CST applicants was 505.15. The cut-off for the 2022–2023 cycle was approximately 513. Preliminary data suggests the cut-off for the 2023–2024 cycle has increased to around 530, although at the time of writing this book this has not been formally verified.

Chapter 3

The Portfolio

3.1 Overview of the Portfolio

Currently 30% of Overall Marks

The portfolio is a collection of evidence demonstrating the applicant's skills, experiences, and achievements as deemed relevant to a surgical career. The portfolio scoring often changes year on year – sometimes substantially. As such, we will not go into great depth about the portfolio, for fear of it becoming out-dated quicky. Instead, information about this can be readily obtained online. All changes are announced on the Health Education England (HEE) website. It will be covered here as a brief overview.

The typical domains include demonstrating a commitment to surgery, teaching and teaching training, research (presentations and posters), and audit and quality improvement projects. While daunting to look at, most marks are achievable in a 6–12 month timeframe if you are motivated and efficient.

Each year the portfolio causes a great deal of stress for candidates – we know it certainly did for us. Do not fall into the trap of thinking you must work non-stop to max out your score. These are unhealthy aspirations and can get in the way of you enjoying your foundation training as well as your life outside of work. If you are sensible and savvy you can reliably secure a strong portfolio score. We list a few tips for the portfolio below.

3.2 General Advice for the Portfolio

Points:Time Ratio

The most important concept to be aware of is the idea of a points:time ratio. Organising a teaching course can be done in around three months with a couple of hours work each week. That would get you the maximum score of 10 points for that section of your portfolio (for the 2022–2023 cycle). On the other hand, completing a PG Cert in medical education will take you anywhere between 6 and 12 months, dedicating roughly 10 hours of work per week (not to mention typically costing many thousands of pounds), all for an additional two points on top of what is achievable in a two-day teaching course. Similarly, for the 2022–2023 cycle, you get the same (full) marks for a two-cycle audit ensuring that venous thromboembolism prophylaxis assessments are performed on your ward as you do for a five-cycle multisite audit on warfarin prescriptions across 2,000 patients. Unless you have a particular interest in warfarin prescriptions, or the project will get you something else like a publication, from a CST application perspective there is no benefit to the more onerous project.

Your time is valuable, and pursuing the most 'high yield' of the portfolio options should be your top priority, where the most points are available for the least number of hours of work. When taking on a project for your portfolio, take a moment to really think about if it's the right thing for you to do. Do you really have the time to commit to this right now? Are there better things you could be spending your time on? Starting a project is a lot easier than finishing one.

Improve your points:time ratio by 'doubling up' projects. For example, run a teaching course with an alternative spin on it – maybe the way you are delivering it is unique, or it is covering a topic that is rarely covered. Write up your teaching course and submit it to a medical education conference – if you can get an oral presentation out of it, then you have nearly maxed out your presentations and publications section as well. The less time spent jumping through hoops for the portfolio the better.

Make a Group

Hopefully you will know at least a couple of people who are going through the application process at the same time as you. Most likely they will need similar things to you. Make a team and split the work. Running a teaching course with two colleagues will massively reduce your workload. Work on three audits, with each of you leading on one of them. Each audit will take one-third the time, and by the end of it you will be the first author on an audit, and a secondary author on two further audits. Your colleagues will bring different skills to the table which will potentially make the projects go further than if you were doing them by yourself.

Bit by Bit

Little and often is the key. Most projects fail because momentum runs out before you can get them across the line. Taking things step by step and committing to doing a few hours a week on portfolio projects will help keep things ticking along until completion. Having said that, if you can't manage a few hours a week, that's fine. It can be difficult to make time for these things, so don't beat yourself up if you're not hitting your self-imposed targets. Keep perspective and keep trucking.

Proof

Each year points are lost by candidates not having the correct proof of their achievements. The HEE website clearly specifies what is required as proof. Read this meticulously and draft a letter for your supervisors to sign off which includes exactly what is required. These letters may look contrived, but you must not put yourself at risk of not getting the full points score you deserve.

Portfolio Scores

What score do you need to be competitive? Naturally, this will vary year on year. Whereas previously there was a 'cut-off' that candidates needed to achieve to get an interview, the MSRA is now used for shortlisting, so the portfolio is simply used to gain additional marks for your ranking.

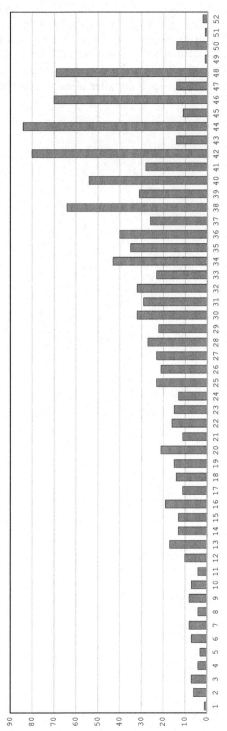

Figure 3.1 Distribution of number of interview candidates (y-axis) with a given verified portfolio scores (x-axis) for the 2022–2023 CST application cycle.
Data obtained via Freedom of Information Act request to Health Education England 24 July 2022, FOI-2307-2006479 NHSE:0176379. © Crown copyright, reproduced under the Open Government Licence.

Data obtained by a Freedom of Information Act request to HEE show that the average verified portfolio score was 33.49/52 in the 2022–2023 cycle. Only around 10–15 candidates scored >48/52. What is interesting to note when looking at the 2022–2023 portfolio score distribution, is that while there is some bunching in the region of 34–48/52, almost 500 candidates scored under 34, with around 90 candidates scoring <10/52 (Figure 3.1). This may be partly due to an influx of candidates who are applying for CST as a second-choice specialty after already completing the MSRA for their first-choice speciality.

Approaching the CST Interview

4.1 Overview of the Interview

The interview is the final stage of your application and includes:

- One three-minute pre-prepared oral presentation on a question usually focused on some aspect of your experience of leadership. This is followed by two minutes of general questions about leadership and management.
- One five-minute management (or ethical) scenario.
- Two five-minute clinical scenarios

This accounts for 60% of your total mark, and with a wide distribution of marks available, this is the main determinant of your final rank. The mark-scheme at the time of writing is listed below.

Every sub-domain below is marked out of 6:

0. No evidence
1. Very poor
2. Weak
3. Satisfactory
4. Good
5. Excellent
6. Outstanding

For 2022–2023, each station was marked by two examiners, who each give a mark out of 6 for each subdomain. The subdomains for each station are:

Presentation:
- Content
- Presentation skills
- Questioning

Management station:
- Probity, professional integrity, and awareness of safety & ethics
- Judgement under pressure & prioritisation
- Communication

Clinical stations 1 and 2:
- Clinical skills & knowledge

– Judgement under pressure & prioritisation
– Communication

These give a maximum total score of 144 for the interview. It is worth noting that communication skills represent a third of the available marks in each domain – 48/144 marks are not for what you say but how you say it. Going from 'good' to 'outstanding' in these categories with both interviewers would boost your mark by a whopping 16 points – marks you will not be awarded if you do not communicate well, no matter what you know clinically.

Data obtained via a Freedom of Information Act request to HEE shows that for the 2022–2023 cycle, the average marks in each station were as follows:

1. Presentation: 27.72/36
2. Management/Ethics: 27.73/36
3. Clinical: 54.81/72

Total = 110.26/144.

The distribution of marks is shown in Figure 4.1. When you consider that the interview represents 60% of your total score, you can see how the relatively large variability in interview scores is typically going to be the single biggest determinant of which job a candidate will end up with.

4.2 General Advice for Approaching the Interview

Practise, Practise, Practise

There is no substitute for putting in the hours to ensure each part of your interview is as slick as possible. Put in time to learn the theory independently outside of practising with colleagues and come prepared to your practice sessions. Give honest and constructive feedback to your partner, and they will do the same for you. Closer to the time of the actual interview, start asking your senior colleagues to provide mock interviews for you, or to listen to your leadership speech. This is where you want to be interviewed by as many people as possible to get a wide spread of feedback.

Perfect Practice

Practise under exam conditions as often as possible, keeping to interview timings. This will help you get used to the pace of the interview. As the interviews are online, you can record your screen to see exactly what the examiners will see on the day. Identify small things you can change such as maintaining good eye contact, moderating the speed at which you speak and cutting out unnecessary filler words and pauses. You can also ensure that the lighting, camera, and backdrop you have for the interview are optimised.

Choose Your Interview Slot

Interview slots are released by email, and it's a first-come-first-served system to get interview slots. If you can, choose a slot that will give you a day or two off beforehand. Think about how you tend to sleep before these exams and your natural body clock – do you perform better in the morning or the afternoon? Interestingly, a recent study

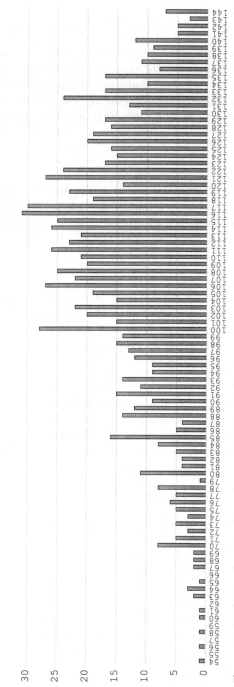

Figure 4.1 Distribution of number of interview candidates (y-axis) who achieved a given interview score (x-axis) for the 2022–2023 CST application cycle.
Data obtained via Freedom of Information Act request to Health Education England 24 July 2022, FOI-2307-2006479 NHSE0176379. © Crown copyright, reproduced under the Open Government Licence.

analysing the 2021 cycle of applicants found that those with morning interviews scored better than those with afternoon interviews, while those with interviews in the second week scored higher than interviews in the first week [1]. It is unclear if this trend is isolated to that year, or if measures have been put in place to address this.

Stay Calm

On the day, you may well get scenarios you have not practised or have interviewers who question you in ways you were not expecting. Just like in all aspects of medicine, this is a test of your ability to stay calm under pressure, go back to the basics, and think logically. The examiners will be trying to get the best out of you – if they jog you about something you have missed, do not panic, they just want to make sure you have covered everything.

Technical Issues

Unfortunately, the nature of online interviews means that there are always going to be technical issues for some candidates. Minimise this risk by ensuring you are somewhere with strong Wi-Fi, and that you have a backup internet supply such as a mobile hotspot ready if you need it.

Interview Courses

These can help to give you a final burst of practice in a more structured way before your interview. However, they are often expensive, and certainly not necessary for everyone, so do not feel pressured to attend one. If choosing a course, ask previous cohorts which ones were useful and carefully assess the proposed faculty.

Resources

A list of essential resources that you should familiarise yourself with before your interview include the ATLS (Advanced Trauma and Life Support) student manual, the CCRISP (Care of the Critically Ill Surgical Patient) manual, RCS guidance on surgical leadership, and up-to-date GMC guidance on key areas as relevant to the management and ethics station.

It Goes Fast

The interview only lasts 20 minutes but will determine to a large extent where you will spend your next two years of training. With the adrenaline coursing through you, it goes by extremely quickly. Be prepared, be confident, and remember to smile.

Outcome

Testing such a small amount of knowledge from such a wide syllabus in such a short space of time will inevitably lead people to feel they have underperformed. Try not to be disheartened if you are unhappy with your score – how you score in your CST interview is not a validation of your ability as a clinician.

Reference

1. Faderani R, Abdi Z, Hastings A, Reed T, Zargaran D, Mosahebi A (2022). 'Core surgical training: The influence of time and date on interview outcome'. *The Surgeon* 21(4): 208–216, https://doi.org/10.1016/j.surge.2022.10.003.

The Presentation

You will enter an online meeting and be greeted by your interview panel. The presentation question will be read to you, and you will be asked to deliver a speech which should be no longer than three minutes. The question varies year by year and can cover broad topics such as leadership, communication skills, and teamworking. However, for several years it has been something along the lines of:

Tell us about your leadership experience and how this could benefit you as a core surgical trainee.

The question is typically sent out a few weeks before the interview to give you time to prepare. When the question is sent out, read it word for word and ensure you answer the specific question they ask. If it is a two- or three-part question, make sure you address all the parts. We will use the question above as a guide for this chapter.

This is the only section of the interview where you are in complete control – you will be allowed to speak uninterrupted for three minutes. This station accounts for 25% of your total marks. You will set the tone for your whole interview in these three minutes. Bear in mind that interviewers will be doing back-to-back interviews all day, often covering very similar ground for each candidate, so standing out with a strong speech is important. You can then carry the momentum of a good speech into the follow-up questions, and the subsequent scenarios.

As part of your preparation ask senior colleagues to share their own successful speeches for your review and ask for feedback on your own speech. We recommend that a few days before the interview you 'lock in' a final draft of your speech and stop making edits and instead cement the final speech in your memory.

Your speech will be graded on three different elements: content, presentation skills, and your response to the interviewers' questions. You will be given a mark out of 6 for each.

5.1 Content

Your task (for the question above) is to create an engaging speech that answers the question in hand while highlighting your relevant experience for CST. There is no one formula for how to write a speech, and speeches that vary in style, structure, and content can all achieve full marks. A speech put together creatively or interestingly will quickly stand out to examiners who hear dozens of speeches each day. When presented with your question, the first step is to break it down and consider what parts you need to answer. For the mock question listed above, it is really asking three separate questions:

1. How do you define the term leadership?
2. What personal experience of leadership do you have?
3. How does your experience relate to your role as a future surgical trainee?

To answer the questions above you would need to read around the topic of leadership and think about what makes a good leader. The Royal College of Surgeons has a short guide entitled 'Surgical Leadership' [1] which outlines what makes a capable surgical leader and the pitfalls of poor leadership. Understanding what leadership entails will help you to identify which of your experiences best animate the themes of surgical leadership.

You would then need to reflect on your leadership experience. This does not need to be related to surgery but should be reasonably recent. In your speech, ensure you demonstrate the impact you had in these roles with specific figures and outcomes. For example, 'I led 5 colleagues to design and implement a 6-session teaching programme for 20 students' has far more impact than saying 'I led a team that conducted teaching sessions.'

It is important to give all parts of the question equal consideration. For example, how your leadership experience relates to the core life of a surgical trainee should not only be referenced in the conclusion. It would be better to return to this theme throughout your speech.

Finally, avoid an over-reliance on buzzwords. Instead, let your real-life experience and passion for the subject come through in your speech.

5.2 Structure

When structuring your speech, we would recommend that you keep broadly to an introduction, body, and conclusion. Or in other words tell them what you're going to tell them, tell them, then tell them what you told them, making it easy for a listener to understand and absorb your key points. The introduction can outline what traits of leadership you will be exploring in your speech, or it could start off immediately with a story that hooks the listener in. A three-minute speech would typically be enough time for two to three short sections on different examples or roles you have held.

You should design your speech so it falls around 15 seconds under the maximum time allocated to ensure you are able to get through it all on the day even if you make a mistake.

5.3 Delivery

Presenting a speech is difficult under pressure. Many candidates will vary their tone, volume, rhythm, and pace inappropriately. Here is where feedback from your peers, recording yourself, and simulating the interview conditions during practice sessions, is important. Around your interview you should be aiming to repeat this to as many people as possible – it only takes three minutes.

When you are practicing with others, the quality of your feedback will influence the quality of theirs. Giving direct and honest feedback will encourage people to do the same to you. Here, we lay out a few elements for a 'mark scheme' on presenting skills to prompt better feedback with colleagues:

- Pronunciation and grammar – are words pronounced correctly? Grammatical errors have no place in a pre-written speech.
- Enunciation – are all words spoken clearly?
- Use of vocabulary – is jargon limited? Is a broader vocabulary demonstrated without using words inappropriately?

- Breathing – is this controlled, and taken at appropriate points in speech? Are they running out of breath?
- Fluency – do they hesitate, repeat themselves, or have unplanned pauses?
- Volume – is an appropriate, consistent volume achieved?
- Pace – do they speak too quickly/slowly? Does the speech overrun? Is the pace consistent throughout?
- Tone and engagement – is emphasis placed on appropriate points/words? Do they effectively engage and maintain interest? Are they suitably enthusiastic about their topics?
- Body language – do they smile appropriately, maintain eye contact with the camera, and use appropriate gestures?

As a tick-box exercise, you should ensure your set-up for a virtual interview is appropriate: lighting, background, camera resolution, camera position, acoustics, microphone quality, and distance from the camera.

By thinking about these different areas when you practise, they will become second nature to you, and you shouldn't need to think about them on the day.

5.4 Example Speeches

Whilst preparing for the interview, we found it helpful to review speeches from previous candidates. The following speeches are based off speeches which scored full marks at the interview. We should stress the scripts below were only part of the equation, and all these speeches were delivered well on the day, were thoroughly rehearsed, and were written to fit with the rhythm and habits of the candidate's natural speech. The speeches have been edited to keep them anonymised, but we have kept the tone and structure the same.

Example 1

My experiences of leadership thus far have shown me that a good leader should be adaptable, organised, supportive, and proactive.

At university, I [was involved in a play]. One night, a cast member felt unwell a few hours before the show. Here, I had to be adaptable, rejigging several key scenes to allow other actors to cross-cover the part, allowing the show to go ahead. This also required keeping the team calm, being decisive, and thinking quickly under pressure, all important attributes of a surgeon.

The project, with its logistics and funding, required me to be organised, and I developed time management skills. I took these with me throughout medical school, helping me [obtain an academic achievement] despite a number of extracurricular projects. I have taken these skills further into my clinical practice, and I organise my time, prioritise my jobs, and complete tasks promptly, all key attributes of a good team player.

As a regional lead in a data collection project, I organised [a team of students] to collect data at multiple hospital sites. I communicated clearly and delegated appropriately, but I made sure I was approachable and supportive by checking in with the teams and having regular feedback meetings. This approach allowed me to identify a struggling medical student early, and facilitate giving them extra support and training, to allow them to continue with the project. It was a great success, and the study was subsequently published in [an academic journal]. As a core trainee, you may manage a diverse group of people, and fostering a supportive working environment is vital in getting the most out of your team.

Finally, as an FY1, it was proactivity that led me to identify that around 5% of our acute medical take was for alcohol-related pathology, but my hospital lacked any sort of alcohol management framework and didn't use CIWA scoring. I formed a team, delegated tasks based on people's skillsets, and came up with a range of interventions, such as CIWA scoring training modules for the nurses, new alcohol management guidelines, and most importantly, getting my F1 cohort engaged to push the changes across the line. The hospital now has a full alcohol management pathway, which I'm very proud of.

Whether it's reading up around operations before attending theatre lists, or developing your surgical skills in your own time, surgical training relies on the trainee being proactive – things aren't handed to you on a plate. I believe that my proactivity, organisational skills, supportive personality, and adaptability will put me in good stead for the rest of my surgical career.

Analysis

This speech followed a common template. It opens with a one-sentence explanation of the core features of leadership, which signposts the traits that will be demonstrated throughout the speech. It involved an extracurricular, academic, and clinical example of leadership. Each section then begins with a brief description of a problem/scenario, followed by how they showed leadership in that situation and finally ties this to the leadership traits of a surgeon. The speech gives the impression of someone who understands the traits of clinical leadership, has considered how this relates to their own experiences, and has thought carefully about which of the traits of leadership they feel are important to core surgical training.

Example 2

Good morning,

I'd like to talk about my experience of leadership as captain of the University volleyball team, and how the lessons I learnt from this will make me a better core surgical trainee.

I have represented the volleyball team throughout my six years at [medical school] and captained the volleyball team during my final year. Volleyball is exceptionally pressurised with the team's success heavily scrutinised. Moreover, players are keenly invested in their place on the team.

My role as captain required me to provide effective leadership in ensuring in-game success, and show empathy in managing emotions outside the game. I particularly thrived when taking personal responsibility for my role in the team, encouraging my teammates to produce their collective best and to troubleshoot pragmatically in the heat of the moment. Fairness and clear communication were fundamental to my approach.

This role also introduced me to some of the less enjoyable, but equally important, organisational aspects of leadership. As captain, I organised transport to away games and managed the team bank account. I improved my time management and task delegation skills from this experience.

After a run of three years of second-place finishes, I'm proud to say we won the regional championship in my final year as captain. I have learnt from the pressures of both winning and losing Championship games; the former highlighting the value of team morale and unity of purpose (as well as some luck!), and the latter illustrating the importance of maintaining perspective and facing up to individual and collective criticism.

Given the academic pressures I simultaneously faced each year, this was a hugely challenging experience. Nevertheless, the teamworking and leadership skills I acquired are transferable to many walks of life, not least to being an effective core surgical trainee.

As a CST, I will use these communication skills to advocate for my patients, motivate and support my team members, and clearly and concisely hand over clinical information. I will also rely on my decision-making skills – assimilating and prioritising information and weighing up pros and cons in emergency situations.

I hope to continue to develop these leadership skills of good communication and clear decision making, to contribute to excellent patient care during my Core Surgical Training.

Analysis

This speech is entirely non-clinical and focuses on a single example of leadership that many candidates will be able to relate to. It does not follow the classic template outlined in this chapter. It stands out due to its clarity, clear understanding of fundamental leadership traits, and sincerity and authenticity. It produces examples of leadership along the way and then reminds you of them when circling back to talk about how it relates to CST.

Example 3

All doctors work in some capacity as leaders and team members.

As a core trainee, this will include working as part of a multi-disciplinary team, supporting more junior colleagues, and participating in organisational change. In my current role as a [teaching fellow] in a [medical school], I co-manage a team of 20 fellows varying in clinical grade from F3 to post-CCT. My responsibilities include rota management, recruitment, and co-ordinating projects, including recently a series of revision sessions on clinical anatomy. The wider team for the project included diverse clinicians and academics and I endeavoured to ensure everyone felt heard, valued, and respected. I used my negotiating skills when scheduling the programme and tried to lead by example in ensuring teaching materials were ready by agreed deadlines.

This experience working in diverse teams will be useful working in the MDT as a core trainee, where negotiation is often important to resolve conflicts. The revision programme received overwhelmingly positive student feedback which I presented to the faculty and GMC representatives. One of the most rewarding aspects of my role has been mentoring medical students. I have sought to emulate consultants who have mentored me, aiming to encourage my tutees to problem-solve themselves, using issues like difficulty engaging as educational opportunities. This complements my clinical experience supporting F1 doctors involved in the [surgery] team, and I hope to continue to support near-peer clinical colleagues as a core trainee.

I have also led change in my organisation, for example, during my F2 [specialty] rotation, when I proposed an audit on my own initiative to assess [whether a test was being ordered according to guidelines]. I recruited a small team of junior doctors, ensuring I was upfront about the expected commitment and time scale. I co-ordinated data collection on almost 1,000 patients, finding [the results of the audit], and this project led to local guideline change projected to save the trust 1,000 pounds per year. It was crucial to ensure the project methodology was communicated clearly and responsibilities were effectively delegated to avoid errors and duplication. These skills are relevant to core training where clinical tasks must be clearly delegated and reflect my desire to continue active involvement in QI and audit leadership.

I hope to continue to develop as a leader and team member as a core trainee, recognising the difference high-quality clinical leadership can make to patient care.

Analysis

This speech uses concrete measures of impact (numerical evidence such as the exact amount of money saved by the trust) to make the answer more impactful. It focuses on the actions and roles of the individual, and when it describes a team, it refers to their specific leadership roles within that team and the actions they personally took.

5.5 Follow-up Questions

Follow-up questions might cover areas in your speech that require clarification or elaboration, or be a range of generic questions about the nature of leadership/teamwork/communication and how these relate to surgery. These can be very broad questions making it extremely difficult to think of a concise answer (of around one minute) on the spot. It is therefore essential you have practised them to prevent yourself from rambling. Prepare model answers for these with example situations that can be easily applied to multiple questions. You need to be able to summarise the background to the role/situation/event/anecdote that you talk about in just a few lines. In preparing this way, you will be forced to think about your leadership and communication skills, which in turn may benefit your presentation.

1. What makes a good leader?
2. What makes a poor leader?
3. Does every member of the team have the same role?
4. What is the difference between leadership and management?
5. How can you maintain high standards of leadership?
6. What different leadership styles do you know?
7. Can leadership be learned?
8. What do you find difficult about leadership?
9. Tell us about a time you had to make a difficult leadership decision.
10. Tell us about a time your leadership was challenged.
11. Are all surgeons/CSTs expected to be leaders?
12. Are you a good team player?
13. Tell us about a time you played a key role in a team.
14. Tell us about a time you helped a struggling teammate.
15. What are communication skills?
16. When have your communication skills improved an outcome for a patient?
17. Tell us about a time you felt you did not communicate well.
18. Tell us about a time you had to deal with a difficult colleague/patient.

It is also worth preparing some more generic broad questions so you are not blindsided by these if they come up:

1. Why surgery?
2. What skills do you have that will make you a good surgeon?
3. What is your greatest achievement?
4. What is your biggest weakness?
5. Tell us about a time you worked well under pressure.
6. Tell us about a time you were out of your comfort zone.
7. Tell us about a time you had to think laterally to solve a problem at work.
8. Tell us about a mistake you have made at work.

Reference

1. Royal College of Surgeons (2018). 'Surgical leadership: A guide to best practice'. Online guide on The Royal College of Surgeons Website, accessed 19 Feb. 2004, www.rcseng.ac.uk/standards-and-research/standards-and-guidance/good-practice-guides/leadership/.

Introduction to the Management Station

6

6.1 Overview of the Management Station

The CST interview includes one five-minute management or ethical scenario. As with the clinical scenarios, you are given a vignette with a question posed at the end of it. After talking through this question, you will be given a number of follow-up questions. This station tests your ability to understand non-clinical problems that arise in the workplace, often centred around key ethical principles such as capacity, confidentiality, and patient safety. These are scenarios that a core surgical trainee might reasonably find themselves in.

The scenarios give you the opportunity to demonstrate you understand the dynamics of working in a team, and that you are an empathetic, sensitive, and honest clinician. The range of possible scenarios is large, so the chance of you having practised the exact scenario is relatively small. However, there are common themes and sub-themes between many different scenarios. Furthermore, there are 'correct' responses to specific issues that you should incorporate into your answer.

There are three elements to preparing for this station. As always, the first is to have a solid foundation of a well-rehearsed structure that can be used in almost any scenario. We will walk you through the 'I-SPIES-DR' framework, which with practice can be used to tackle almost any case.

The second is to revise the basic guidance, facts and pathways we cover throughout the cases. This revision will centre upon common GMC guidance and key legal issues encountered in medicine. Reading this information and then practising how to articulate it succinctly is essential.

The third element is to hone your judgement by regularly practising scenarios. With repetition, you will find it easier to identify the common themes that are being tested in a scenario and have a better understanding of the actions you need to take. You will build up a repertoire of actions to take in these scenarios that demonstrate you have integrity, are conscientious, and know how to reflect on your actions. We have offered model answers, but these are by no means the 'only' answers. As you practise outside of the pressure of the interview, take time to think of any other positive actions you might take for each scenario. This will provide you with tailored, authentic responses to situations which will help you stand out.

Put all three elements together: a robust structured approach to a scenario, understanding the key legal and ethical frameworks for given situations, and regular practice putting those two together, and you can score highly in this station. Do not fall into the trap of thinking this is a soft station that you can coast through – it is worth 25% of the interview marks and through practice you can increase your score significantly in a relatively short space of time.

6.2 Framework to Approach the Management Station

It is important to have a consistent structure that you can fall back on at the start of the scenario. Having a framework that you are comfortable with will help stop you from missing the obvious points, while providing you with more breathing space to think of points tailored to the specific scenario in question.

The framework we used was the 'I-SPIES-DR' approach:

I – Issue

– What is the main issue or issues that this scenario is asking about? Highlighting the key issue(s) is a good way to introduce your answer. Some of the most common issues in these cases include patient safety, honesty/integrity/probity, communication, teamwork, bullying, prioritisation, fairness, consent, capacity, confidentiality, and the duty of candour.
– If the issue is not immediately obvious to you then you can skip this – it may become more apparent as you talk through the scenario.

S – Seek information

– It is important you gather all available information. Demonstrate you are being conscientious, methodical and not simply jumping to conclusions.

P – Patient safety

– Highlighting the possible risks to patient safety is your next priority. In the (few) scenarios where there really are no risks to patient safety then you might reference this by saying: *although there are no direct risks to patient safety, this behaviour is still concerning due to. . .*

I – Initiative

– It is vital that you show you are attempting to manage the situation to the level that is appropriate for your grade. It is unhelpful and unrealistic to immediately escalate everything to your senior.

E – Escalate

– As with the clinical scenarios, escalation up the chain of command is likely to be required. The route of escalation should be appropriate for the scenario and occur in a logical stepwise fashion.
– Whom to escalate to depends on the scenario, but consider your educational/clinical supervisors (ES/CS), the consultant on call, the departmental clinical director, the hospital medical director, the site manager, the training program director (TPD), your medical defence organisation, your union, occupational health, your GP, and counselling services.

S – Support

– Support your patients: consider how they have been affected and how you as a doctor can help them.
– Support your colleagues: this may be through helping them yourself if appropriate or signposting them to get help from other people. It may involve simple things like being flexible and swapping shifts.

- Support your department: being flexible with covering shifts and helping with rota changes if required. Organising audits and teaching are useful ways to share learning points with your team.
- Support yourself: through reflecting, but also through formal support via your CS/ES, occupational health, and your GP. Acknowledging that some scenarios may be profoundly stressful is important, as is knowing how to get help for yourself when required.
- Think about who in each scenario needs support – you won't need to say all four in every case.

D – Document
- Any scenario in which there is an error in care or a near miss should be reported through an incident reporting system (Datix). Most scenarios should be documented in some fashion – be that through a Datix, in the patient's notes or through your logbook/portfolio.

R – Reflect
- This is a way to support yourself. Avoid a throwaway line such as *I would reflect on this* – use it to demonstrate you understand the severity of the situation. Think about what you are reflecting on and why. Consider reflecting with your supervisor, writing an account of the event (especially when there is any concern about medicolegal fallout) and reflecting privately in your logbook/portfolio. Using online training to improve the skill assessed in the scenario is another way to reflect actively.
- If you have identified a systemic structural issue, consider performing an audit to quantify the problem, or organising teaching to help address it. This is a form of reflection and a way of supporting your team and patients going forward.

It is worth pointing out that most candidates will be entering these scenarios with some kind of framework. As a result, it is likely the examiners will be hearing an iteration of roughly the same script for most applicants. This is not necessarily a bad thing – a confident, smooth and logical answer that addresses all the issues in the scenario and demonstrates that you are a kind, sensitive trainee should be enough to get you full marks.

However, you should avoid the temptation that a framework brings to hear a buzzword (e.g. 'a struggling colleague') and set off down a formulaic path. You must address the specific details provided in the scenario. Confidence in your framework will free up brain space to allow you to take stock and think of specific extra points for the scenario to help you stand out as a thoughtful and considerate colleague. This will also help you to avoid sounding unnatural and robotic, which is a risk for candidates who stick too rigidly to their framework. Similarly, not every part of the framework is needed for each scenario, and trying to shoe-horn points in will look forced. With practice you will become more confident excluding unnecessary sections from your responses.

Cases will initially be written out verbatim *in italics* to provide a feel for how the cases should sound overall, but as the cases progress, short-form responses will be provided to allow you to develop these into full answers of your own. Answers will intermittently revert to the verbatim style throughout the chapter to keep reminding candidates of the structure and flow of a full model answer. Follow-up questions are provided after the case, which will aim to cover some of the common ethical and legal principles. In some cases, we also provide similar scenarios to think about, which are iterations on the same theme, that you can practise with a colleague.

Management Scenarios

7.1 Lost Notes

You are a general surgical CT1 and are conducting an audit of VTE prescriptions on your ward. You have taken the paper notes for several patients home with you to work on that evening. When you get home you realise you have lost your backpack, containing the notes, on your journey home. How do you proceed?

Issues

This scenario raises serious issues around patient confidentiality, data security, and patient safety, as well as the duty of candour.

Seek Information

To begin with, I would identify what notes were lost, at what time, for which patients, and if there were electronic backups.

Patient Safety

If the notes were not immediately found there is a clear patient safety issue which must be addressed. Patients rely on their right to confidentiality when seeking medical help, and private health-related information being made public may put patients in a vulnerable position. If the notes are lost without a backup this may also disrupt continuity of care.

Initiative

In the first instance, I would retrace my steps to see if I could find the notes. I would consider calling a colleague who is still at work to see if they can check common areas such as the changing rooms or doctors' mess for my bag and consider calling the public transport company if I used this to get home.

Escalate

Given the severity of the situation, it's vital that I escalate this – most likely to the consultant in charge of the patients or to my educational or clinical supervisor. I will need senior support in addressing this issue. I would also escalate this to the data protection champion or Caldicott guardian for my trust. It may be worth alerting my medical defence organisation to the situation as well. If there is an archival backup, then escalating to medical archives and ensuring a replacement copy of the notes is available to clinical teams caring for the patient is a priority.

Support

In accordance with the duty of candour, I would arrange to discuss the situation with the affected patients (ideally face to face) to apologise and explain what happened, how it is a breach of standards, how it may affect them going forward, and what we are doing to put it right. I would ensure that electronic backups were located, which may involve contacting the patients' GPs for their community notes. I would ensure that the relevant specialties looking after the patient are aware of the problem to prevent issues with continuity of care. I would consider if there was a lack of clear guidance about this issue, and if I can arrange further teaching on safe handling of patient information for my wider team. It is also important that I support myself in this time – I would acknowledge this is going to be a stressful period for me and ensure I am being open about whether I need more support at work.

Document/Reflect

It is vital that a Datix is reported for this incident. Given that this is a serious lapse in judgement it would be prudent to reflect in my portfolio about what I have learnt from this. I would complete e-learning on patient confidentiality and data protection. I would review GMC guidelines and reflect with my educational supervisor about what prompted my lapse in judgement and how my subsequent response could have been improved.

What is the duty of candour and what GMC guidance is provided for this?

The duty of candour is a statutory duty described in GMC Good Medical Practice [1]. It determines that doctors must be open and honest with patients when things go wrong. GMC guidance notes that in situations where something has gone wrong, you must:

1. *Tell the person when something has gone wrong.*
2. *Apologise to the person.*
3. *Offer an appropriate remedy or support to put matters right (if possible).*
4. *Explain fully to the person the likely short- and long-term effects of what has happened.*

What legislation is relevant to patient data?

The Data Protection Act (1988) governs the protection of personal information. For example, as little information as needed should be stored for as little time as possible and this information should be stored in a secure way (such as using encryption on a memory stick). Moreover, information must be used fairly and lawfully. The act also gives individuals the ability to request access to their information. The GMC has produced guidelines on 'good practice in handling patient information' [2].

In what instances is it acceptable to breach patient confidentiality?

A number of instances exist where it is acceptable to breach patient confidentiality. For example, when discussing with other healthcare team members information which is relevant to the patient's care, when ordered to do so by a court order, necessary disclosure to a statutory body such as GMC, when required in the public interest such as for notifiable diseases or the prevention of death or serious harm to other individuals, or in cases where patients who lack capacity are experiencing, or at risk of, abuse or neglect.

References

1.   General Medical Council (2018). 'Openness and honesty when things go wrong: The professional duty of candour'. Website, Gmc-uk.org, www.gmc-uk.org/ethical-guidance/ethical-guidance-for-doctors/candour—openness-and-honesty-when-things-go-wrong.

2.   General Medical Council (2018). 'Confidentiality: Good practice in handling patient information'. Website, Gmc-uk.org, www.gmc-uk.org/ethical-guidance/ethical-guidance-for-doctors/confidentiality.

7.2 Colleague Incapacitated at Work

You are a plastic surgery CT2 assisting on a registrar-led skin cancer list. Your registrar comes to morning handover acting erratically, trembling, and sweating. His pupils are noticeably dilated. When you ask him if he is feeling well, he says that he has 'had a late night'. How do you proceed?

Issues

The most important issue in this case is patient safety – there are signs indicating my registrar may be under the influence of drugs and is therefore unfit to operate effectively or be in a clinical environment. Another important issue is professionalism, as coming to work in such a state is clearly unacceptable. I would also consider my colleague's wellbeing – coming in to work intoxicated may be indicative of problems in their personal life.

Seek Information

I would take my registrar to one side and ask them directly, but in a non-confrontational way, if they are under the influence of drugs. It is worth noting that I would need to act even if my registrar denies drug use, as from the information provided to me, I have clear concerns that this is the case.

Initiative

After asking my colleague directly, I would explain my concerns about patient safety, and explain to them that they need to return home. I would check to make sure they have a safe method of transport home as driving home is clearly inappropriate (and illegal) in this case.

Escalate

At this point I would escalate the situation to a suitable senior colleague – likely the consultant on call or the consultant in charge of the skin cancer list. I would do so with discretion; whatever the outcome from today, this will be an immensely difficult time for my colleague, and gossiping will not help anyone. The consultant will both be able to help arrange cover for the operation list and follow the situation up – it is not my role as a junior doctor to investigate my colleague's home life or drug-taking habits.

Support

There are several groups who need to be supported in this situation. First and foremost, I would support my patients by ensuring they understood there may be a delay in their operation.

I would avoid telling the patient the exact reason why this has happened – this would likely undermine the confidence of these patients in the profession and involve jumping to conclusions before an appropriate investigation has been carried out. If pressed, I would say that the operating surgeon is not well. If cover cannot be found, I would make sure the patients were safely booked in within an appropriate timeframe to return for another operation.

I would support my colleague by being non-confrontational, avoiding gossiping, and offering to support my colleague if they are having a difficult time. I would signpost them to occupational health or counselling services in the hospital. I would support my team by ensuring I was flexible with helping out where needed and ensuring cross-cover is arranged to maintain safe staffing levels.

Document/Reflect
I would complete Datix to ensure this incident is formally logged. I would organise a meeting with my educational supervisor to discuss how I handled the situation, and anything I might have done better. I could document this meeting as part of my reflection in my portfolio. Writing a contemporaneous account will also be useful in the event of any ongoing investigation. It is a stressful experience, and my supervisor can be a source of support and guidance.

Your colleague agrees to go home but asks you to not escalate it further and to just tell the team he is unwell. He assures you this is a one-off that will not happen again. How do you proceed?
While telling my colleagues he is unwell is a good approach to avoid gossiping, I would reiterate I must still raise the issue with a supervising consultant. I would be empathetic but firm and stress that it is better to resolve this through proper channels to ensure he gets the support he needs. This is in both his and the patients' interests longer term. It is worth noting from my point of view that if I were to say nothing and a future incident occurs where patients come to harm, it is indefensible for me not to have raised concerns at an earlier point. Moreover, his actions raise probity concerns as he is trying to implicate me in covering up his behaviour – this will also need to be reported.

N.B. if the interviewers press you on this point, you must remain steadfast that you would always escalate to the consultant.

Additional Scenarios to Practise
Consultant coming into work incapacitated
Escalate to the consultant on call and the clinical director (in charge of all consultants in the department).

Registrar is not currently incapacitated, but a bag of white powder falls out of his pocket
Note the uncertainty in this situation – is this a drug, are they using it, are they selling it? Assess for current patient safety risks and escalate this to someone who is more appropriate to investigate.

Colleague watching child pornography at work
Seek information – be clear about what you saw, could it be a mistake or a pop-up? This is illegal, and your colleague may not be safe to be around vulnerable patients – prompt

escalation and removal of colleague from clinical environment in the interim is needed. It should not be up to you to call the police. Contemporaneous documentation is vital here.

7.3 Bullying and Harassment

You are the CT1 on an orthopaedic ward. During the ward round, one of the consultants makes multiple sexist comments to a female F1, referring to her as 'sweetheart', and commenting that the skirt she is wearing will 'make all the patients feel better'. You are aware that patients have witnessed the interactions. How do you proceed?

Issues

The most important issues in this case are bullying, harassment, and maintaining patient trust in the profession. This is bullying behaviour, and the comments about her physical appearance constitute sexual harassment. We know from the 2023 study by the Working Party on Sexual Misconduct in Surgery that two-thirds of women in surgery have been the target of sexual harassment from colleagues in the past five years [1]. This highlights how prevalent such behaviour is, and these actions must not be tolerated.

Seek Information

I already have sufficient information about what has happened but would wait until after the ward round to address this, away from patients.

Patient Safety

It's important to bear in mind that this is indirectly a patient safety issue; disruptive and bullying behaviour is a major cause of adverse events in the NHS. Moreover, if patients have witnessed these interactions, it may damage their trust in the profession.

Initiative

After the ward round I would take the initiative to speak to the affected colleague. I would do so in private, away from patients and other colleagues. I would acknowledge the unacceptable behaviour, see how it affected them, and discuss how they would like to take the situation forward. It would be useful to understand if this is the first time this has happened. I would offer to accompany my colleague to speak to the consultant, although I would be guided by my colleague's wishes – they may prefer to raise this concern through another channel. I would make sure the colleague felt happy to continue patient work today and would offer to manage their clinical work as appropriate to allow them to have a break if needed.

If speaking directly to the consultant, then it must be explained why what they have said is not acceptable. This should be done in as non-confrontational way as possible. However, GMC guidance is clear that we have a duty to challenge colleagues who are not treating other colleagues with respect.

Escalate

This behaviour is unacceptable and should be escalated. Again, I would be guided by how my colleague wants to proceed, and could help them raise these issues together, or signpost them to the relevant pathways. There may be local trust policies in place regarding bullying, but typically the pathway may include their clinical or educational supervisor, the clinical director, the HR department, the anti-bullying lead, and the Freedom to Speak Up Guardian for the trust. I could also approach any consultant that my colleague or I have a good relationship with to help. In the first instance, it may be necessary to structure the rota such that the victim and consultant do not share clinical duties for the time being.

Support

I would support my colleague by checking in with them regularly, at what may be a stressful time – particularly if there is an ongoing escalation process or the issue is not fully resolved. I would signpost them to other sources of support including the BMA bullying service. I would also want to apologise to any patients for what they witnessed.

Document/Reflect

I would ensure I had written a clear contemporaneous account of the events – this can help with reflecting on what happened and will also be important if there is going to be some form of investigation into the incident. It would be useful if any colleagues who also witnessed the events did the same. To better my understanding of this area, I could consider reading some of the growing body of literature around bullying and gender-based discrimination in surgery. Bystander training, which is offered by some NHS trusts, would also be useful to equip me with further skills to address these behaviours in the future.

Additional Scenarios to Practise

Colleague does not want to take it further

Respect their wishes regarding how the situation is managed. You need to balance this with a duty to challenge these behaviours – this can be done outside the context of this immediate instance but should still be done. Seeking advice from a senior colleague on how to balance these two requirements would be prudent.

Consultant shouts at you during ward round

Shouting at someone is unacceptable, but the level of escalation the situation requires should vary based on your understanding of the consultant. If it is a one-off incident, the consultant is contrite, and you know there were unusual triggering stressors that day, how you respond should be different to if this is bullying behaviour that happens daily. Nonetheless, these scenarios are largely predicated on challenging the behaviour where possible and escalating appropriately.

Reference

1. Begeny CT, Arshad H, Cuming T, Dhariwal DK, Fisher RA, Franklin MD, Jackson PC, McLachlan GM, Searle RH, Newlands C (November 2023). 'Sexual harassment, sexual assault and rape by colleagues in the surgical workforce, and how women and men are living different realities: Observational study using NHS population-derived weights'. British Journal of Surgery 110(11): 1518–1526, https://doi.org/10.1093/bjs/znad242.

7.4 Distressed Colleague

You are an ENT CT1 in a busy head and neck department. One afternoon you find your F1 colleague crying in the doctors' office. You know they have been struggling to adjust to the ward; they often stay late, they appear flustered during ward rounds, and the pharmacist has picked up on several small prescribing mistakes they have made. How do you proceed?

Issues

This scenario raises a number of issues. First and foremost is my colleague's welfare. Adjusting to life on a busy ward can be tough, and difficulties at work may also be a manifestation of problems in other aspects of their personal life. Secondly, there is a patient safety issue to address, as several small prescribing issues have been noted.

Seek Information

To begin with, I would want to gather more information. If able to, I would hand my bleep to another colleague, find a quiet side room and then sensitively and non-judgementally ask how my colleague is doing. I would want to check first if they are happy to talk to me about it – it may be there are people they would feel more comfortable talking to. I would explore if there were particular stressors that the team could help with – for example, understaffing, a lack of senior support, a lack of training in specific things like electronic prescribing, a difficult colleague, or if there are issues at home. Identifying the cause will help determine how I approach the scenario.

Patient Safety

Before doing this, I would want to ensure there are no urgent jobs that need doing on the ward that would take priority. Mistakes with prescribing, while minor, may be a precursor to a more serious incident, and so must be addressed.

Initiative

I would then see how I could help cover work in the short term – if I can help with urgent tasks on the wards, swapping shifts, or arranging extra support or cover. I would assess if there were structural issues that need addressing, such as an understaffed rota. As a more senior trainee, it may be easier for me to approach the rota coordinator and explain the issue on their behalf. I would consider if there was any further teaching that I could provide. I would support them on personal issues as best I can but would signpost them to relevant resources such as occupational health, their GP, and counselling services who may be better placed to do this. I would also need to ensure the issue of prescribing errors is brought up with my colleague (either by myself or their supervisor). However, this will need to be done sensitively, and can happen after this initial discussion about their welfare.

Escalate

If I feel that my colleague's welfare or prescribing errors are putting patient safety at risk, then we have a duty to escalate this, most likely to their educational or clinical supervisor.

This must be done constructively, and I would frame this as helping them to get the support they need. If possible, I would encourage my colleague to raise it with their supervisor themself. If I had to raise it myself, I would not do this without letting my colleague know, as this may damage our future working relationship.

Support

It is essential that I, and the rest of the team, support my colleague through this. Our colleagues are human beings and personal issues can interfere with work; having an understanding and supportive working environment can make a big difference, as can signposting to other sources of support. I would help support my team by being flexible with swapping shifts to help arrange cover if the colleague needs some time off.

Document/Reflect

I would document the steps we had taken to address any prescribing errors. If any further errors were identified that resulted in patient harm then we would have a duty of candour to the patients.

It's important that I reflect on this event myself – we are all fallible and there may be times when similar issues happen to me. I would think about what my own coping mechanisms are for these situations, and what my support network would be if I needed to share these concerns at work.

Additional Scenarios to Practise

A number of different scenarios may be the pretext for a struggling colleague – persistent prescribing errors, persistently turning up late, or taking regular sick days. Make sure patients are safe and then ensure your colleague is being supported holistically.

7.5 Refusing to Treat a Patient

You are the general surgical CT1 helping run an outpatient general surgical clinic. Your registrar refuses to see the next patient, who has a previous conviction for child sex abuses. How do you proceed?

Issues

The key issues in this case are patient safety, the patient's right to care, the wellbeing of a colleague, professionalism, and the GMC guidance on refusal to treat a patient.

Seek Information

To begin with, I want to gently explore my colleague's reasoning for their actions. It is important to understand if my colleague feels directly threatened by this specific patient (from a previous encounter or due to their behaviour in the waiting room, for example) or if my colleague is refusing on principle to treat them due to their history as a child sex offender. I would also check if anything similar to this has happened to my colleague before, and how it was managed then. I would check for any local protocols applicable to this situation.

Patient Safety

It is essential that I ensure the patient is stable and there are no pressing clinical concerns while this is being resolved. The patient has the right to receive the same standard of care regardless of their conviction and this care should be delivered by someone whose behaviour is not affected by their beliefs. Given the strength of these beliefs from my registrar, it may not be appropriate for them to see this patient.

Initiative

I would take the initiative and act within my own competency to help the patient, including seeing them myself if appropriate. Otherwise, I would find a suitable senior who can see them, such as the consultant in charge of the clinic, or other registrars who are available in clinic.

Escalate

I would want to discretely inform the supervising consultant of the situation, and going forward this may need to be discussed with the registrar's clinical supervisor, who would be best placed to support the registrar on this matter. They may need to arrange a meeting to discuss their beliefs, and ensure they are aware of the GMC's advice on this issue. If my colleague is refusing to see this patient in principle due to their conviction, this may be in breach of their duties as a doctor. If a patient is not being abusive or threatening, there are few instances where doctors have a statutory right to conscientiously object to treating a patient.

Support

Throughout this, I would ensure the patient is supported to get the treatment they need. By resolving this matter promptly we will also be helping the other patients in the department by ensuring the smooth running of the clinic. I would ensure my colleague is supported; most doctors would not refuse to treat a patient without very good reason, so I would be sensitive to what may be a distressing experience for them.

Document/Reflect

This is a complex scenario and reading around the GMC's and BMA's guidance around refusal to treat patients would be prudent. I could consider delivering departmental teaching on this topic but must ensure this is balanced with supporting my colleague and ensuring suitable discretion regarding the incident. I would want to reflect on this situation with my own supervisor to see if there were ways I might have managed the situation better.

Additional Scenarios to Practise

'Refusal to treat' scenarios can manifest in many situations, such as managing a racist or aggressive patient, or in situations involving conscientious objections to treatments. The questions below will clarify some of these areas. You should have senior support in any situation where care is potentially being denied to a patient.

Are there situations in which doctors can conscientiously object to certain procedures? What should doctors do in these situations?
The GMC acknowledges that doctors have a right to their own personal beliefs and can conscientiously object to providing care which conflicts with their sincerely held beliefs and moral concerns. However, a conscientious objection may not be based on self-interest or discrimination. Moreover, you may only conscientiously object if it does not deny patients access to appropriate medical treatment. Therefore, you cannot object to providing emergency care.

If you have a conscientious objection to a particular procedure, you must explain this to the patient and explain they have a right to see another doctor – if it is not practical for the patient to arrange to see another doctor, you must ensure a suitably qualified colleague is able to take over the case. In doing so you must not show disapproval about the patient's choice. This is covered in some detail in the GMCs 'personal beliefs and medical practice' document [1].

Note there are few areas where doctors have a statutory right to conscientiously object. The most important area where this is relevant is around abortion – specifically that doctors can conscientiously object to providing the termination of pregnancy as per Section 4 of the Abortion Act 1967. Note this does not apply in an emergency, and nor does it apply to care before or after the procedure.

Do abusive patients have a right to care?
Patients always have a right to emergency treatment (provided it can be given safely). Patients also have a conditional right to non-emergency care. Healthcare workers have the right to work in an environment free from abuse, harassment, and discrimination. This potential contradiction was clarified in 2019 when the GMC confirmed its position was aligned to that of the BMA. They noted that in a situation where a doctor refused care appropriately, professionally, and in line with local procedures and BMA/GMC guidance, to a patient who was abusive and who did not need urgent care, that doctor would be well positioned to justify their actions if required [2].

What should you do if a patient refuses to see a doctor of a particular ethnicity?
Patients have a right to request a particular doctor if they have a reasonable reason for the request. If a patient refuses to see a colleague based on their ethnicity, this may amount to them refusing care. Remember that in situations where (non-emergency) care is potentially being refused to a patient, it is essential you have senior support to guide you.

BMA guidance on this topic advises you to engage with the patient, determine why they are making a discriminatory request, and explain that this is unacceptable behaviour, and that these requests cannot be accommodated [2]. If the patient removes their request, then confirm with the colleague in question that they are still happy to continue providing care for the patient. If they do not remove their request, then explain this will impact their ability to seek care at this organisation and explain their rights to seek care at another organisation. Document clearly their refusal to withdraw their request, and that the patient understands the risks, benefits, and alternatives to their request. The patient cannot be forced to be treated by a doctor they refuse, but they cannot demand a doctor of a particular ethnicity.

References

1. GMC (n.d.). 'Personal beliefs and medical practice'. Website, accessed 19 Feb. 2024, www.gmc-uk.org/ethical-guidance/ ethical-guidance-for-doctors/personal-beliefs-and-medical-practice/personal-beliefs-and-medical-practice.

2. British Medical Association (2022). 'How to manage discrimination from patients and their guardians/relatives'. Website, www.bma.org.uk/media/5144/bma-guidance-on-how-to-deal-with-discrimination-from-patients-march-2022.pdf.

7.6 Audit and Clinical Governance

You are the CT1 on general surgery, you notice that your patients are often not being correctly prescribed VTE prophylaxis on admission. You decide to undertake a project to improve this. How might you identify whether this is a persistent problem in the department, and what could you do to improve this?

N.B. this scenario does not fit into the I-SPIES-DR framework and is unlikely to be your standalone management scenario. However, a good understanding of this case will help with many common follow-up questions.

The scenario presented raises patient safety concerns, as a failure to correctly prescribe VTE prophylaxis will result in avoidable VTEs and direct patient harm. I would want to systematically assess how the department is performing on this subject in relation to national guidelines. This would be best assessed using an audit.

The stages of an audit are to identify an issue and a relevant gold standard such as a national guideline. I would talk to a suitable consultant who would be able to provide supervision and guidance for the project and register the audit with the appropriate team at the hospital. I would then collect data using a systematic approach to ensure a suitable sample of patients are included. This will likely involve retrospective case note analysis from recent inpatient admissions. I would compare our practice to the gold standards and present the results back to the wider team – a local clinical governance meeting would provide the perfect forum for this. We would then discuss suitable interventions to help address this, such as teaching on the topic (which I could help organise), an easier pathway at the hospital (e.g. putting this on an admission proforma), or a way of regularly checking this (e.g. making checking VTE a part of the ward round proforma). I would ensure that the whole MDT was engaged in this plan-in this case the nursing staff and pharmacists will have important roles to play. I would then reaudit the data after a pre-specified time to determine if these interventions had an effect and report these results back to the team. I would consider what further changes could be made for another cycle of the audit and consider delayed cycles to determine if the interventions have had a lasting effect.

What is the difference between an audit and a quality improvement project?
The key difference between the two is that the audit has a gold standard, against which performance is measured. A quality improvement project would be better suited for a project aiming to, for example, increase staff wellbeing – for which there is no clear national standard.

Why are audits important?
Audit represents one of the seven pillars of clinical governance, and the GMC guidance on 'Good Medical Practice' recommends doctors should take part in regular audit of current

practice. These will ultimately ensure we are delivering a high standard of care for our patients. For trainees such as myself, audits provide the opportunity for junior staff to understand service provision and national standards, while also providing an opportunity to present projects to colleagues locally, or through conferences.

What issues have you found with audits you have performed?
Performing powerful audits to high standards takes time, and it can be difficult to achieve when regularly rotating through departments. Moreover, it can be frustrating when retrospective data is limited by things such as poor documentation, as this can limit the impact of your findings.

What is clinical governance?
Clinical governance is an umbrella term describing a range of processes by which we maintain and improve the quality of care that patients receive, while also ensuring there is accountability of the system to patients. It is built on the seven pillars of clinical governance (PIRATES):

- *Patient and public involvement: patients are involved in the monitoring of outcomes and the development of our clinical services. For example, the use of PALS to engage with patient concerns.*
- *Information and IT: data is used to measure clinical outcomes, and that data is treated respectfully.*
- *Risk management: learning from mistakes and near misses. Critical incident forms are key in this.*
- *Audit: to ensure that practice is monitored and areas to improve are identified.*
- *Training and education: supporting lifelong learning to keep up with the advancing medical field.*
- *Effectiveness and research: using evidence-based medicine and altering our practice based on the latest evidence while contributing to research to enhance future care of patients.*
- *Staffing and site management: appropriate recruiting and management of staff including good working conditions.*

You would not be expected to list all the pillars of clinical governance in this format. It is worthwhile to have examples for two or three of the pillars above to show your experience of clinical governance. Teaching programs, critical incident reports, research projects, and audits that you have been involved in would all be useful here. Being able to describe the scope and outcomes of a project you have been involved with in two to three lines is essential and should be practised.

7.7 Aggressive Patient

You are the urology CT1 reviewing a man with epididymo-orchitis in the emergency department. It has been extremely busy, and the patient has waited five hours to see the emergency department team, and then four hours to see yourself. He is clinically well. He is frustrated by the wait and irritated at having to repeat parts of the history to yourself after already telling the emergency department team. He is becoming abusive and begins to shout. How do you proceed?

Issues

This scenario raises a number of issues. The first is my own personal safety – in any situation that may turn violent, my first priority must be to ensure my own safety and that of other members of staff. In theory, there is also a potential risk to other patients in the department. Abusive behaviour is all too common in the NHS, and verbally abusing a staff member is completely unacceptable and must be acted on. Finally, the scenario highlights a nine-hour wait to access a specialty assessment – this may point to systemic issues within the department regarding support and staffing that may need addressing.

Seek Information

After confirming that the patient remains clinically well (as a deteriorating clinical state could cause delirium and aggression), I would need to make a judgment about whether I felt immediately at risk or not. If I did, I would calmly walk away and get help – the nurse in charge of the emergency department would be a good person to speak to initially as they will have experience of how to manage these situations, which may require getting security involved.

Initiative

If I felt that I was not in danger, I would engage the patient calmly and attempt to verbally de-escalate the situation. I would still ensure that the patient was never between me and the door, and that I re-evaluated if the threat of violence changed. I would give the patient my undivided attention (passing my bleep to a colleague if I was able to) and conduct the conversation in a quiet space or side room. I would keep a neutral stance, speak calmly and slowly, and make sure the patient felt listened to. The patient has been waiting a long time and may be in pain or discomfort. I would acknowledge this, explain why it has been the case, apologise on behalf of the department, and ensure I had offered the patient analgesia if needed. I would explain why I am having to take a history a second time, as it's important that I get the facts right in my own head to perform a proper assessment, and ensure no details have been missed.

Escalate

How the consultation would go from there will depend on how the patient responds to my attempts to de-escalate. If I felt I was not able to de-escalate, I would excuse myself and discuss the situation with my senior colleagues – likely the registrar on call in the first instance. Having a more senior member of the team talk to the patient may help calm them down, and they may need to take over the consultation if I felt that my relationship with the patient was unrecoverable. It is essential that it is explained to the patient that abusive behaviour is unacceptable and will not be tolerated, and a failure to change their behaviour may result in them being asked to leave. Ideally, this should be explained in such a way as to avoid further inflaming the situation. It is essential to escalate up the chain of command if you are considering asking a patient to leave, and to involve security if required to ensure that this is done safely. Different units may have different local protocols (e.g. a 'yellow card, red card' system) for these situations which you should follow.

Support

Once the situation was resolved, I would ensure that I had apologised to patients nearby for what they may have overheard, as this may have upset other people. I would ensure I received suitable support myself – being shouted at by a patient can be extremely upsetting, and debriefing properly with a colleague can go a long way to helping process this. I would consider discussing the situation with my supervisor after the event, with whose help I might be able to analyse how to approach the scenario better in future.

Document/Reflect

I would meticulously document the encounter with objective facts, times, and verbatim text where possible, particularly in any situation where a patient is asked to leave the department. I would also submit a Datix – my employer has a duty to protect staff from discrimination or harassment, and there may be learning points they can take forward to help prevent this in the future. Finally, it is important to assess why the patient had such a long wait to see me – was it a particularly busy day, or is this a regular occurrence? Do the SHOs need more senior support? Auditing the time from emergency department referral to urology assessment and presenting these findings at the next clinical governance meeting would be helpful for the department and would serve as a good catalyst to discuss interventions which may help if there is a systemic problem.

How would the scenario change if you were assessing an acutely aggressive multi-morbid elderly gentleman who has cognitive impairment on the ward?
I would be particularly vigilant to the possibility that this patient may have become acutely confused, contributing to his aggression. An A–E with a confusion screen should be undertaken if there are any concerns about this. I would attempt to use the least restrictive method to control the situation and prevent harm to the patient, myself or any other patient.

N.B. the 'aggressive patient' scenario may come up by itself, or as part of a follow-up question to many scenarios involving patient communication, so it is important to have this prepared. The key principles will revolve around managing risk to the safety of staff members and escalating abusive behaviours appropriately. BMA guidance here is very useful [1].

Reference

1. British Medical Association (2022). 'How to manage discrimination from patients and their guardians/relatives'. Website, www.bma.org.uk/media/5144/bma-guidance-on-how-to-deal-with-discrimination-from-patients-march-2022.pdf.

7.8 Consent and Capacity

You are the vascular surgery SHO. A woman admitted yesterday is on the ward awaiting an urgent lower leg amputation for a gangrenous limb. On the day of the operation the patient, who was consented for the procedure yesterday, withdraws her consent and refuses to proceed with the amputation. She is withdrawn and irritable when you go and speak to her.

Issues

- Consent and capacity: it is a legal requirement that patients who have the capacity to consent have their wishes respected. Equally, patients lacking capacity must be managed appropriately through the Mental Capacity Act.
- Patient safety: the patient has a gangrenous limb, and the apparent change in their cognition may represent a worsening of their underlying clinical condition, such as in the context of delirium.

Seek Information

- You should first ensure the patient is clinically stable using an A–E approach. There are many reasons why they may have changed their mind, but you must rule out the possibility that they have clinically deteriorated, and this is affecting their decision making.
- Explore with the patient their decision making and why they have changed their mind. Ensure they fully understand the procedure in question, the indications, and the likely outcomes from other management options.

Patient Safety

- You have asesssed to ensure the patient remains clinically stable. If concerned they are deteriorating, manage these in an A–E fashion escalating to your seniors as appropriate (this is not a clinical case, so do not start describing a full operative workup).

Initiative

- Assess their capacity to make this decision at this moment in time. As per the Mental Capacity Act, this involves assessing whether the patient can understand, retain, and weigh up the information you have provided, and then communicate their decision to you. Remember that all patients are presumed to have capacity until it is formally assessed for that specific decision.
- If you are unclear about their capacity, your senior should review the patient, and you should seek advice from other members of the team involved in their care and get input from their next of kin about their baseline cognition and any ways to enhance their ability to make a decision beyond clinical optimisation.

The interviewer interjects: you perform a capacity assessment and deem that the patient lacks the capacity to consent for this operation, how do you proceed?
The issues and patient safety concerns in this situation remain similar, and given this is a potentially life-threatening situation, it is worth escalating to your seniors early and keeping the operating team updated on the situation. If content that they do not have capacity, you should determine if the patient can reasonably be expected to regain capacity in an acceptable timeframe – in which case you may be able to delay the decision making if clinically safe to do so.

In the scenario where they are unlikely to regain capacity without treatment, you must first find out if they have a valid advanced directive regarding treatment. In this situation, the advance directive must specifically mention the risk of death without treatment to be applicable. If it is not valid or legally binding, it may still be useful later as an indicator of the patient's wishes. Next you must identify anyone with lasting power of attorney (LPA), this must specifically be an LPA for matters relating to health. They can legally make decisions on behalf of the patient, and you should provide them the relevant information to inform their decision as you would for a patient. If neither of these exist, then a best interest decision will need to be made by the clinical team on behalf of the patient. A best interest multi-disciplinary team may be convened to do so, involving the doctors, nurses and other clinical staff. Input from previously expressed views of the patient when they had capacity (even if not legally binding), and family members should be considered. You should always consider which management option will be the least restrictive option to their future choices, particularly if they may regain capacity in future.

The interviewer interrupts: the patient has no advance directives or Lasting Power of Attorney (LPA) and you cannot get hold of their family. They are continuing to deteriorate and need to go to theatre immediately. How do you proceed?
Treatment in this situation is preventing potential loss of life or serious deterioration in health. The clinical team can therefore treat the patient in their best interests, completing a consent form 4. In situations where serious medical treatment is involved, if there is no legal proxy or person close to the patient who can represent the patient then you should instruct an Independent Mental Capacity Advocate (IMCA) who can help represent a patient's interests.

Document/Reflect
-   Your documentation should be rigorous, showing all options and avenues explored, the full breadth of information gathered and the reasons for the eventual decision. You must document a formal capacity assessment, and any measures taken to ensure the patient was given the best chance to regain capacity. You must show you took reasonable steps to locate an advance directive or LPA. Your justification for a best interest decision should be based on multisource evidence and show why you believe it aligns with the patient's views, values, and priorities.

Can an LPA refuse life-saving treatment on behalf of a patient?
Yes, but this must be specified clearly on the LPA form. If this happens, it's essential you explore their reasoning and ensure they fully understand the risks and benefits of the treatment programs. Senior input would be essential, and input from the hospital's legal department may be advisable. Advance care plans or LPAs that do not specifically mention life-saving treatment should still be consulted, even if they are not legally binding for this procedure, as they will contain important information to help guide the final best interest decision.

What criteria exist for consent to be valid?
Valid consent must be given by someone who has the capacity to make that decision, it must be given voluntarily, and it must be informed consent – that is, based on appropriate and correct information.

Can patients with capacity decline medical interventions even if this will result in death?

Yes. Autonomy is one of the four pillars of medical ethics. If the patient has capacity, it is both immoral and illegal to then subject them to treatment they have refused. They should be given all the relevant information about the potential consequences of the decision. The information and the patient's responses should be carefully documented.

If members of the MDT disagree about a best interest decision, what could be done to resolve the disagreement?

As per the GMC guidance, local resolution is preferred. Options include consulting more experienced colleagues, involving an independent advocate, holding a case conference or using the clinical ethics committee at the trust. Thereafter, formal policy and legal steps should be followed to resolve disagreement.

Reference

1.   GMC (n.d.). 'Decision making and consent'. Professional Standards – GMC, Website, accessed 19 Feb. 2024, www.gmc-uk.org/professional-standards/professional-standards-for-doctors/decision-making-and-consent.

7.9 Never Event

You are the plastic surgery CT2 running a local anaesthetic skin list. Your registrar is in the theatre office next door, and you are performing the list independently. You have recently removed a lesion on an elderly man's right forearm and the patient is now back on the ward. While writing the operation note, you realise the patient had been consented for removal of a skin lesion on the left forearm. How do you proceed?

Issues

–   Never event: wrong site surgery is a never event and must be dealt with as such. There are multi-step processes in place to ensure wrong site surgeries do not occur, and a failure of these processes to prevent this represents a serious breach of care standards.
–   Patient safety: the patient is post-op, so their immediate clinical safety must not be forgotten. Moreover, a potentially dangerous skin lesion on left forearm still needs to be dealt with.
–   Duty of candour: a mistake has been made and this must be raised with the patient.

Seek Information

–   Confirm the patient details, check what operation they were expecting, check the clinic letters, consent form, the side the patient was marked, and the preoperative documentation and WHO checklist. Determine at what stage the mistake was made.
–   If there was an error only in the consenting process and technically the 'correct' side was operated on, it is still a serious issue – the patient was consented for a different procedure. This still represents a failure to properly conduct the WHO safety surgical checklist.

Patient Safety

- Assuming the patient was stable when he left the theatre, there is no immediate risk to patient safety. However, the need for another procedure has associated risks and can increase morbidity.
- The patient may be less likely to seek help in the future for skin lesions due to a loss of trust. It is therefore even more important that you handle the situation transparently and tactfully from this point onwards.

Initiative

- Alert the registrar/consultant in charge of the list to what has happened.
- Go and speak to the patient to explain what has happened. As per the GMC duty of candour you must offer an apology, explain what happened, explain the likely short- and long-term effects, and explain what you are doing to right the situation. This will result in an internal investigation, the results of which will be presented to the department via the clinical governance process. It would be prudent to go with your senior to the patient for this discussion.
- You should emphasise to the patient that you will work to ensure this does not happen to any patients in future. You might offer to provide the patient an update on the outcomes of any investigation and the measures put in place, thereafter.
- Give the patient time to process what has happened, be available to discuss this again with the patient later in the day if required or speak to family over the phone if they wish.
- Offer the patient the opportunity to speak to your senior.
- Offer the patient the opportunity to raise a complaint by giving the contact details for PALS. You should emphasise that using this service will not affect their care.
- Discuss with the bookings team to determine when the second operation will be.

Escalate

- The severity of this incident means you have escalated to your senior immediately. This is something you should raise with your educational supervisor as it will require further investigation. It may also be worth contacting the BMA/your defence union.

Support

- The patient: ensure they are safe following the first operation, and that they have suitable follow-up booked to remove the correct lesion.
- Your department: be proactive in helping with whatever patient workup is needed for a new operation (assuming the patient is happy for you to be involved in their care going forward).
- Your theatre colleagues: a major mistake has been made at some point in the preoperative process, and the members of the theatre team that day will therefore be involved. Ensure you have a proper debrief and see if any errors in your conduct can be identified.

- Yourself: being directly involved in a never-event like this will be stressful, and ensuring your support mechanisms are in place is important.

Document/Reflect
- Write a contemporaneous account of what has happened in the patient notes. This should be thorough and detailed to facilitate further investigations.
- Submit a Datix for this instance. This will require a full investigation under NHS England's Serious Incident Framework, the findings of which should be presented at the relevant clinical governance meeting.
- Consider if more teaching on safety protocols is required.
- It would be prudent to reflect with your supervisor on this instance who can guide you as to how the incident will be managed going forward.

What are never-events?
A list of pre-defined preventable serious patient safety incidents that should never happen. The NHS publishes and updates a list online of these specific events. The ones most likely to relate to surgery include wrong site surgery, wrong implant/prosthesis, and retained foreign object post-procedure (e.g. a retained swab).

Can the patient request another team to take over their clinical care?
Patients have a right to request another clinician provided this is for a justifiable reason – this situation would be justifiable. Ensure you have been honest and have apologised. See if the patient would be happy to continue with your team but without your specific involvement. If required, facilitate the transfer of care to a suitable team with a detailed handover.

What is the WHO surgical safety checklist?
The WHO checklist is a standardised set of safety checks for surgical teams to undertake before any operation. A brief summary of the steps are offered below:
- Sign in (before the induction of anaesthesia): confirm identity, the site (marked), and the surgical procedure. Check for allergies, confirm if there is a difficult airway, aspiration risk and risk of blood loss.
- Time out (before knife to skin): confirm identity, site (marked), procedure, sterility of instruments, and that relevant imaging is displayed, and essential safety steps considered.
- Sign out (before the patient leaves theatre): Confirm procedure, complete instrument/sharps/swabs count, discuss any equipment issues and concerns for postoperative care.

There are two extra steps in the 'five steps to safer surgery', produced by the Royal College of Surgeons. These are a briefing before the list to introduce staff and address any concerns for the list and a debrief at the end of the day to evaluate the list and discuss any learning points.

What is a Datix?
A formal incident reporting system that is used in many NHS trusts. These are usually accessible through the trust's intranet. The reporting of errors in care or near misses is

one of the pillars of clinical governance, and these reports are then investigated with a root cause analysis to see what can be learnt from them.

What other common ways are there for incidents to be reported and discussed, and for changes to be made?
Audits and QIPs are important avenues to implement and demonstrate positive changes. Morbidity and mortality meetings are another avenue within a department to learn from incidents. The local clinical governance meetings provide a good opportunity to present and discuss all of these findings.

Additional Scenarios to Practice

You realise on-table that the patient has been consented for wrong surgical site. The patient has been put to sleep, but no incision has been made yet
Wake the patient up – do not proceed with a possible wrong site surgery. When awake, a similar protocol to that described above can be followed. You may reference local operating theatre procedures for your trust, but it is crucial that you do not attempt to proceed.

7.10 CEPOD Negotiation

You are the on-call general surgical CT1. One of your patients, who is septic due to a perianal abscess, is due to be operated on as the next case on the emergency operating theatre (CEPOD) list. You are bleeped by the plastic surgery consultant asking if their case – a replant of a 9-year-old's finger – can go ahead of your patient. How do you proceed?

Issues

- Patient safety: two patients who require immediate (life- or limb-saving) operations.
- Communication: between two specialties, the theatre staff, theatre coordinator, and anaesthetic team.

Seek Information

- A great deal of information is needed to resolve this situation. You need to know how unwell each patient is. In the case of the finger, is this injury part of a polytrauma case where other injuries need to be managed as well? Are both patients fully 'ready' for surgery – are both on site, checked in, do they both have any necessary preoperative workup, blood results, group and saves? Are they consented, marked, and starved, and have an appropriate postoperative bed to go to? Are both operating teams fully ready or do other members of the team need to come in? How long does each team expect their case to take? Does either patient need further resuscitation before coming to theatre? Is any special equipment needed for the cases (e.g. microsurgical kit for the replant) and is this kit ready and available?

Patient Safety

- Regularly re-reviewing your patient with ongoing resuscitation will be essential while this process is ongoing to ensure they are not clinically deteriorating, which may also influence the discussion around operative planning.

Initiative

- Alert the theatre coordinator, bed manager, anaesthetic team, and theatre teams to the potential clash. Alert your senior to the situation – the decision will ultimately rest with the consultants on call.
- Explore other options that may help to resolve this, such as opening another theatre, or 'breaking into' an elective list that is already running that day. Are there patient flow issues through theatres which could be ameliorated by promptly discharging other patients under your team's care?

Escalate

- Decisions about critical operation planning such as these are consultant-led decisions, and in the event of difficulty agreeing, the relevant consultants on call will need to speak directly.
- If all local resolution options fail and both teams feel their case cannot be delayed further, then the final option is transfer of one patient (blue light ambulance) to another site or trust that can perform the operation. However, the steps of consultant-to-consultant discussion, opening another theatre, or using an ongoing list are typically sufficient.

Support

- Your patient: your patient is septic and will need ongoing reviews and resuscitation while these discussions are taking place. It is also important to keep them updated (and possibly their next of kin) on the progress of the situation as they will no doubt be anxious to have their operation as quickly as possible.

Document/Reflect

- Discussions with other specialties should all be documented in the patient's notes.
- Auditing whether patients are meeting national criteria for timings of emergency operation would be a useful metric to determine if there are systemic issues with emergency theatre availability. These concerns can be escalated up and may result in more CEPOD theatres being opened.

What is NCEPOD?

The "National Confidential Enquiry into Perioperative Deaths" (NCEPOD) was a report from the 1980s looking at the factors contributing to perioperative mortality. Over time it has come to refer to emergency surgical procedures, or the theatre where these cases are performed. The report found that overnight operating increased the risk of perioperative death.

The CEPOD classification is shown in Table 7.1.

Table 7.1 CEPOD classification with example cases and expected timeframe

Category	Examples	Timescale
1: Immediate *1a life saving* *1b limb saving*	Ruptured AAA Testicular torsion	Ongoing resuscitation with surgery, to be performed within minutes. Break into other operating lists if needed.
2: Urgent *Life, limb, or organ* *threatening*	Strangulated hernia Critical limb ischaemia	Within hours; use emergency list in and out of hours.
3: Expedited *Stable patient requiring early* *intervention*	Tendon and nerve injuries	Within days; use elective lists with 'spare' capacity or daytime emergency list.
4: Elective *Planned procedures booked* *in advance with routine* *hospital admissions*	All conditions that are none of the above categories	Planned.

What is ASA grade?

Developed by the American Society of Anaesthesiologists (ASA), the system grades patients and is validated for quantifying the risk of death under anaesthetic.

ASA I: normal healthy patient.

ASA II: mild systemic disease such as well controlled-hypertension or diabetes, and smokers.

ASA III: severe systemic disease such as poorly controlled diabetes, BMI > 40, or end-stage renal disease on dialysis.

ASA IV: severe systemic disease that is a constant threat to life such as a recent (<3 months) myocardial infarction, shock, or sepsis.

ASA V: a moribund patient not expected to survive without the operation such as a ruptured abdominal aortic aneurysm.

ASA VI: a patient declared brain dead whose organs are removed for transplant purposes.

Some limitations to the system include the lack of age as a marker, although this is known to impact operative mortality, and the grey area between grades II and III for patients with stable disease of a moderate nature.

7.11 Managing a Patient against Guidelines

You are the plastic surgery CT1 on a ward round with your consultant. Your consultant notes a patch of cellulitis on a patient's leg and advises you to start co-amoxiclav and metronidazole for this. You know that the recommended antibiotic on local guidelines is flucloxacillin and you raise this with your consultant, who insists that she has 'seen this before' and states that co-amoxiclav and metronidazole is better in these situations, before moving on to the next patient. How do you proceed?

Issues

- Patient safety: a patient is getting broader spectrum/ incorrect antibiotics. This may subject the patient to antibiotic-related complications that they could have avoided,

as well as failing to target the organism in question sufficiently, while also promoting antibiotics resistance.
- Professionalism: senior doctors should encourage junior colleagues to speak up about patient safety issues, and not dismiss them, to foster an open environment.

Seek Information
- It is vital that you are correct in your interpretation of the guidelines, so check these again. Remember that guidelines are there to guide clinicians to making the right decision but are supposed to be interpreted in light of the patient in front of them – there may well be a good reason why this guideline isn't being adhered to and it is important not to jump to conclusions.
- Check if there are patient-related factors (such as allergies, severity of infection, previous infection history, or recent swabs) that you have missed.
- Ask the consultant if there are specific guidelines she uses in these situations, or a clinical reason why she has deviated from them – there may be more recent guidelines or evidence that the consultant has used to make this decision.

Patient Safety
- There is a patient safety risk if incorrect antibiotics are prescribed. There is also a patient safety risk in general when doctors fail to take on board pertinent advice.

Initiative
- Once satisfied that there are not good reasons for this management, it is important you act: if the consultant is doing something you feel to be unsafe, you must raise this with them.
- The timing of your action is important – ideally this can wait until after the ward round and be away from the patient's bedside. However, if there is a risk the wrong antibiotic will be given imminently, then this discussion should be had now.
- You can politely raise your disagreement by phrasing it as a learning point – wanting to know if there are specific reasons that the consultant has chosen that antibiotic for that particular patient, seeing as it is different to the guidelines. It is important that you preserve your future working relationship.
- Checking with your registrar to see if you are missing anything obvious is helpful. The ward pharmacist would be useful in a disagreement about a specific medication and given this is an antibiotic decision the on-call microbiology team would be well placed to help resolve the issue. Use of an authoritative third party is a non-confrontational way to resolve the issue.

Escalate
- If despite your concerns they continue to do something you feel is unsafe, then it would be appropriate to escalate this. Initially, your registrar will be able to talk to your consultant, but beyond this you would need to speak to the microbiology consultant, the consultant on call, your ES/CS, or the departmental clinical lead. It's important that you only escalate once all avenues to sort this out have been exhausted, as this may have implications for your ongoing working relationship with the consultant.

- Remember that in an emergency, where there is no time to seek another opinion, you would need to let the consultant's decision stand. It is important in this situation you have recorded your disagreement in writing.

Support

- Support your consultant to make the right decision by providing them with correct guidelines, and ensuring the mistake is raised in a polite and respectful way. If this is a recurrent issue you could invite the microbiology team to provide teaching for the department on antimicrobial stewardship and the common antibiotics used in your department.
- Support your patient by raising this promptly to avoid a medication error.
- Support yourself by ensuring disagreements are documented in writing if needed.

Document/Reflect

- Whatever the outcome of this scenario, there will be a useful learning point for you – either how to manage a clinical disagreement, or new management pathways that you had not appreciated. It would be worth reflecting on this in your portfolio.
- Another way to reflect on the event may be to perform an audit of antibiotic prescribing habits within your department. You may have identified a pattern of mistakes that needs addressing, and an audit would be well placed to identify any systematic issues.

What is the difference between a guideline, a protocol, and a standard?

- A guideline provides advice on how to act in a given situation. For example, haematology guidelines on how to manage a suspected VTE in hospital. This guideline is there to guide you by providing you with information in order to make the correct decision for your patient.
- A protocol describes a series of steps to accomplish a set goal. For example, the hospital may have a protocol for ambulating patients with a confirmed VTE.
- A standard describes an acceptable level of quality or attainment. For example, there may be a national standard that all inpatients should have a VTE risk assessment on admission to hospital.

7.12 Rota Dispute

You receive the monthly on-call rota which is put together by one of the CT2s in your department. You can see that for the second month running you are assigned to more time on call and on the wards than your colleague, who has put herself primarily on operating lists. How do you proceed?

Issues

- Probity and professionalism: if your colleague is not acting honestly in designing the rota then this is a serious issue that can affect ongoing trust and teamworking.
- Training: adequate theatre time is required by core trainees to progress in their training and develop as surgeons.
- Patient safety: doing more than your share of on-calls may make you more fatigued and therefore more likely to make mistakes.

Seek Information
- Do not jump to conclusions about what is going on. Ensure you have double checked the rota – asking another colleague to review the rota may be helpful. Check also if you have suitable rest days in place after on-call shifts and that the rota remains compliant with EWTD regulations. Check previous rotas to confirm if there is a pattern – this will provide a larger body of evidence of a trend if needed.

Patient Safety
- As above, if you are fatigued at work, you are more likely to make mistakes. With all rota issues, ensuring safe staffing levels is of paramount importance.

Initiative
- Speak to the colleague who made the rota. It may be a simple oversight that they are happy to rectify. Frame this discussion in a non-confrontational way. See if you can arrange swaps in the short term to ensure the rota is fair while it is being re-figured.
- If you have concerns you are not getting time in theatre, then this should also be discussed with your colleague. It may be that they have highlighted areas they wish to develop to their supervising consultant and as such have been allocated more time in specific theatres and it is simply a case of you doing the same. Concerns about operating exposure should be raised swiftly to ensure there is sufficient time to implement solutions.
- In the meantime, ensure you are progressing your training in other ways, such as using the time on call to practice triaging referrals and performing procedures. Time on call and on the wards will provide plenty of learning points for your training portfolio.

Escalate
- Concerns about probity should be escalated to your ES/CS who can investigate this further.
- Failure to resolve rota disputes can be escalated to medical HR and the departmental consultant leads.
- If there are issues with your training you can escalate these to your ES/CS, then your surgical tutor (an RCS trainee representative for the region), and then to your TPD.
- Ongoing issues regarding contracts and rotas can also be escalated to medical staffing, and the BMA.

Support
- Yourself: ensure you are getting sufficient recovery time between shifts. Ensure you are getting suitable surgical training from your placements, and while these issues are being resolved, take matters into your own hands by attending courses/surgical skills laboratories/practicing at home. It is important you show you can take ownership of your own training and be resourceful.
- The rota coordinator: help them amend the rota. Being a rota coordinator is a laborious and often thankless task that is critical in the safe running of a department – errors and oversights should be managed sympathetically.

Document/Reflect

- If there are consistent issues with the rota or staffing in a department, it is important this is logged in some way so that systemic issues can be identified and resolved. This may be through exception reporting (if you stay late, or if shifts are understaffed) or auditing doctors' hours and the EWTD.

Is probity important?

The GMC highlights probity (acting in a trustworthy and honest manner) as an essential trait for doctors, helping to justify the public's trust in the profession. It is also important to foster good working relationships within the clinical team.

7.13 Late to Handover

You are a general surgery CT1 on call. Evening handover was meant to start 25 minutes ago but the night doctor has not arrived yet and you have had no communications from them. You have an acutely unwell patient on the ward and have been referred a new patient from the emergency department. This is the third time this SHO has been late attending a handover with you.

Issues

- Patient safety: there is an unwell patient and a new emergency department referral, the stability of whom you do not know. They must take priority in this situation.
- Your own safety: you've likely had a long on-call day and need adequate rest before your next shift.
- Professionalism/colleague's wellbeing: the night SHO is 25 minutes late but has failed to communicate with you. This may be concerning for their welfare in the short term. Alternatively, if this is a recurrent problem, a wider professionalism issue may be raised.

Seek Information

- First, call your colleague or try to contact them and find out where they are. Call them, check group chats to see if anyone has heard from them, see if you have the number of a partner or housemate of theirs. Check your own email to see if the rota manager or a consultant has written to inform you that they are unwell or that there is an alternative plan for cover.
- In the interim you are still responsible for the patients, and you should prioritise them based on acuity, so gathering information on them is important, particularly the one in the emergency department who you have not seen. This will also facilitate a faster handover if your colleague arrives.
- Find out what other support and cover is available, including whether a night registrar is on site.

Patient Safety

- If there are acutely unwell patients, these must be reviewed and stabilised urgently. While it is not ideal that you are working beyond your allotted hours, there is no

confirmation of how long the wait for cover will take, and you should continue covering the on call until help arrives.
- You should also be aware of your own deficiencies due to tiredness. Tired doctors make mistakes, so be wary of your own fatigue and do not work beyond a point at which you are too tired. It is unlikely that working an extra 30 minutes after your shift ends would push you into this bracket.

Initiative and Escalate
- While you are awaiting confirmation of the night cover plan, you should review the acutely unwell patient.
- You should escalate the situation to your registrar and then the on-call consultant. You should inform the site manager who will be useful in identifying staff members elsewhere in the hospital who can help with specific duties.
- You could take the initiative to text other SHOs to see if they are able to cover if it is confirmed your colleague is not attending and there is no alternative plan.
- Make a list of all the required jobs and their order of clinical priority to facilitate a quicker handover when it does happen.
- The available options for cover are: hiring a last-minute locum, cross-cover by another specialty, or a senior stepping down to cover the shift. You should not try to cover the full shift as you will have worked too many consecutive hours without a break.
- After the acute incident is resolved, you will need to escalate concerns about repeated lateness to your seniors – discuss this with your ES/CS who can then liaise with your colleague's ES/CS. Do this after the incident so that you have spoken to your colleague, as this will help guide if this is a simple professionalism issue or a more complicated wellbeing one and therefore you will have a better idea of what kind of support your colleague may need. The rota coordinator should be made aware if there are going to be ongoing issues with night staffing.

Support
- Your colleague: remember that while the colleague may be exhibiting an apparent lack of professionalism, there may be an underlying cause that needs addressing and the colleague may need support through this.
- Yourself: make sure you get appropriate rest between shifts. This may mean agreeing a later start the next day or time off in lieu through the on-call consultant or your rota coordinator
- Your patients: continue to care for them until support arrives, prioritise tasks to make handover easier.

Document/Reflect
- Exception reporting is a formal mechanism to report instances where you have had to stay late, through which you can claim overtime pay or time off in lieu. It is important to document this through a formal system, so that systematic trends can be identified, and to help modify staffing levels in the long term.

Additional Scenarios to Practice

There is a recurrent issue with locums cancelling at the last minute

This requires your answer to focus on both the short-term escalation (as above) but also longer-term escalation. This may involve submitting a Datix, escalating to the rota coordinator or the clinical director to ensure appropriate staffing and that repeat offenders are not consistently hired as locums.

7.14 DNACPR

You are the general surgical CT2 on take and have finished clerking in a frail elderly patient with small bowel obstruction. The patient has severe heart failure, poor renal function, and advanced dementia. After discussion with the ITU and anaesthetic consultant on call, your consultant decides that attempting cardiopulmonary resuscitation on the patient would not be appropriate. You are asked to lead the discussion with the family about resuscitation. How do you proceed?

Note: DNACPR decisions are made by senior members of the team, and while discussions with patients and their families are usually led by senior members of the team, it is essential that junior doctors can have these discussions if needed.

Issues

- Communication: this is potentially one of the most difficult conversations a patient and their family can have with medical staff, and it must be dealt with sensitively. It is also important that you feel experienced and able to have these conversations – if not, you should ensure you obtain appropriate training and experience in leading these discussions.

Seek Information

- You must go into this interaction with a thorough understanding of the patient. Read through their admission notes to date, check their recent investigations, and any input from other specialties. It is likely the family will want an update on recent developments, and this can also serve as a natural segue into talking about a treatment plan going forward.
- See if there have already been any discussions regarding resuscitation.

Patient Safety

- Ensure the patient is happy to have this conversation with their relatives present from a confidentiality point of view – remember throughout this scenario that this should be a discussion between yourself and the patient. A diagnosis of dementia does not preclude the patient from being the main partner in these discussions, and whatever their cognitive function, efforts should be made to include them in the discussion as much as possible.

Initiative

- Ensure there are no clinically urgent tasks to complete, and then inform your team that you would like to hand your bleep to someone whilst you go and have the discussion.
- Find a quiet location (e.g. the relatives room/a side room).

- Start by providing an update on their clinical course, recent investigations, and results, and signpost that you are going to talk about planning for if the patient becomes more unwell. Ask what the patient and family understand on the topic of treatment escalation plans, and if they have had any previous discussions about this. At this point some people may volunteer important information about their attitudes to resuscitation. It is important to understand the patient's preferences and values. How the conversation develops will in large part be guided by this.
- Gently explain that the senior clinicians in charge of the patient's care feel that cardiopulmonary resuscitation would not be suitable for the patient.
- It is important to give the patient and their family time and space to air their responses, as well as to highlight concerns or perceptions they have that may need addressing.

It is unlikely you would need to talk through the entire conversation in a station, but important points you could reference if needed would include

- The fact that unfortunately clinically frail patients are significantly less likely to have a positive outcome from CPR, and even in cases where the heart can be restarted, patients may end up with an unacceptable quality of life.
- The reasoning behind the decision and the fact that the medical team are all in agreement that this is in the best interests of the patient given their complex past medical history.
- That decisions are made on a case-by-case basis and are not permanent.
- This decision relates to one specific set of treatments – chest compressions, breathing for the patient, and attempts to restart the heart – and does not affect the other aspects of their care. The decision only takes effect the moment a patient's heart stops beating.
- You will continue to provide the best possible care for the patient regardless of if they have a DNACPR in place or not.
- You may signpost them to online information or provide written information after the conversation.

Escalate
- Explain that these decisions have been made by consultant colleagues and facilitate them having a discussion with your consultant if they would like. It is essential that senior input is obtained whenever it is required for these conversations.

Support
- The patient and their family: empathise with them, give them your undivided attention and offer to come back to discuss any further questions they may have – there is a lot of information to take in, and it's important they have time to process this as this will often yield new questions.

Document/Reflect
- It is vital that a DNACPR form is completed in accordance with local guidelines and that other treating teams, including the GP, and the nursing staff, are aware. This form should indicate that the reasons for DNACPR were explained to the patient

and/or their next of kin. The discussion should also be documented in the patient's notes.

- It is not uncommon for moments like this to affect clinicians – they can be difficult conversations to have. It's important you are in tune with how it has affected you personally, and consider reflecting on this with colleagues, supervisors, and in your portfolio, if you feel it would be beneficial.
- Ideally, all patients who enter hospital should have a treatment escalation plan in place – this is something that could be audited.

The family are adamant that they want their relative to be for CPR – can this be demanded?

As with all medical treatments, the decision to provide it belongs to the medical team, who should not administer treatments which are not felt to be in a patient's best interests. As such CPR cannot be demanded by the family. However, given these discussions relate to the cusp of death, they are significantly more emotive for the people involved. It is therefore even more important that there is some form of consensus between the family and the medical team in this situation if possible. In situations like this the conversation should be led by your seniors, and the presence of seniors from multiple specialties (e.g. anaesthetics and ITU) would be helpful.

Who can put in a DNACPR?

Typically these are put in place by doctors. They usually need to be signed by the senior member of the team in charge of the patient's care – this signature is normally needed within 24 hours.

What is the Tracey Judgement?

Published in 2014, this judgment related to a patient Janet Tracey, who had terminal lung cancer. During an admission for a cervical spine fracture, she had a DNACPR order put in place without this being discussed with her, despite her having capacity and expressing wishes to be involved in all treatment decisions. It was ruled that in doing so the Trust were in breach of Mrs Tracey's human rights. It is now a national standard that doctors should discuss all DNACPR decisions with patients and their next of kin as soon as possible unless there are exceptional circumstances.

How often do patients survive in hospital cardiac arrests?

A question they are unlikely to ask, but may be useful for discussions with patients, as research shows that members of the public typically overestimate the success rate of CPR. Only around a quarter of those treated by the hospital resuscitation team following in-hospital cardiac arrest of all ages will survive to discharge, and of these around a fifth will not have a favourable neurological outcome [1]. Survival rates for older patients are considerably lower than for younger patients.

Reference

1. Resuscitation Council UK (2021). 'Epidemiology of Cardiac Arrest Guidelines'.. Website, www.resus.org.uk/library/2021-resuscitation-guidelines/epidemiology-cardiac-arrest-guidelines.

7.15 Operation Cancelled

You are the general surgical CT2 on call. You clerked in a multi-morbid patient with a perianal abscess who was due to go to CEPOD this afternoon. They are currently stable (albeit in pain), but they require an ITU bed postoperatively. You are called by the ITU bed manager alerting you that there are no ITU beds available, and the patient's operation will need to be delayed until tomorrow. How do you proceed?

Issues

- Patient safety: an undrained perianal abscess may result in sepsis in this multimorbid patient.
- Patient comfort: even if haemodynamically stable the perianal abscess may be causing severe pain.
- ITU capacity and patient flow: consider if there are systemic issues with ITU capacity or patient flow at this unit.

Seek Information

- Clarify which patients are involved, confirm when you expect a bed to be made available, and if there is anyone being stepped down imminently. Confirm if your patient has been fasting, how long they have already been waiting, and if they have already had this operation cancelled before.

Patient Safety

- The most important element in this case. The source of infection is not controlled in a multimorbid patient – re-review the patient and ensure they remain clinically stable. The scenario changes if the patient deteriorates as they will be higher priority for CEPOD and an ITU bed.

Initiative

- Discuss this situation with the theatre coordinator and anaesthetic/scrub teams to make them aware of the situation. It is important the operating team are made aware immediately, and that the named consultant in charge of the patient is aware. Confirm if the patient must have an ITU bed after the operation – could a lower level of care be appropriate? Discuss with the ITU team to confirm there are no imminent stepdowns or extra capacity that can be made available.
- Once you know the above, if the operation is definitely being delayed until tomorrow call the ward immediately and tell them to allow the patient to eat and drink.
- Attend the ward and explain the situation to the patient. Ideally, discuss this in a quiet side room having given your bleep to a colleague temporarily. Apologise on behalf of the team, explain you are working to get this resolved as quickly as possible, and if there is a likely timeframe for getting the operation then give this to the patient. In general, avoid making a definitive promise of a specific date or time (it is unhelpful to do this if you are not absolutely certain it will be stuck to as missing a hard deadline may irritate patients further). Offer to speak to their next of kin if they would like.

- See if there is anything you can do to make the patient more comfortable in the meantime. Make sure the patient has suitable analgesia – perianal abscesses can be extremely painful.

Escalate
- Offer for your senior to discuss this with the patient as well.
- Ensure the situation has been escalated to the consultant in charge of the patient and the bed manager.

Support
- The patient: ensure they are safe, comfortable, and have a plan for ongoing care. If they are unsatisfied and wish to raise a complaint, provide them with the details of PALS.
- The operating teams: you now have an empty space on CEPOD – could this be used for another patient?
- The department: ensure your colleagues are aware of the protocols for booking ITU/HDU beds for postoperative patients.

Document/Reflect
- Document discussions you have with ITU as well as the patient. Ensure they are booked in correctly for the future operation and have an ITU bed for this.
- Send a Datix to log delayed operations – they are potential causes of patient harm, and formally logging this is important for management to get a picture of how frequently this is happening so that resources can be allocated appropriately.
- An audit of this could be performed to determine if this is a recurrent issue.

When telling a patient their operation is cancelled, they become verbally abusive
If possible, this should be managed in a quiet side room with your bleep safely handed to someone to look after for a few minutes. Initially attempt to de-escalate the situation using empathetic active listening and verbal de-escalation techniques. Acknowledge the frustration of waiting for a procedure like this – it may be that they have anxieties about the upcoming procedure that you can explore with them. It's also important to exclude their aggression being due to a deterioration in clinical status. If the patient is continuing to be abusive, this should be escalated to your senior. If there is any danger of physical harm to yourself, you should leave the situation immediately and get help from people like your registrar, the nurse in charge of the ward, and security. Ensure other patients on the ward are safe and not distressed by the outburst. The patient will need to be engaged with to explain why this sort of behaviour is unacceptable and may result in them being unable to seek care at this unit. Raise instances like this in accordance with local policies – your trust will have specific policies for aggressive patients. Moreover, your employer has a duty to protect staff from discrimination or harassment, and there may be learning points they can take forward to help prevent this in the future.

The patient wants to put in a complaint. What is PALS?
All hospitals will have a PALS (Patient Advice and Liaison Service) team who will usually be the first point of contact for patients seeking to feed back on the service they have received. They provide an avenue of support and can liaise directly with the consultant in charge of the patient's care.

7.16 Trauma in a Jehovah's Witness

You are an orthopaedic CT1 and you have been called to a trauma call in resus. A 35-year-old male patient was ejected from a car at high speed and is currently unconscious. They are bleeding from a complex femoral fracture and are becoming progressively more haemodynamically unstable despite aggressive resuscitation. Their haemoglobin is now 65. As you are putting up a unit of blood a family member approaches and says he is a Jehovah's witness and therefore won't want a transfusion. How do you proceed?

Issues
- Capacity and consent: the patient is unable to consent himself.
- Patient safety: the patient is acutely unwell and prompt action is needed.
- Communication with family members and patient's personal beliefs: refusal of a blood transfusion is a core value for some people; going against this can have large implications for a patient.

Seek Information
- Confirm the patient is still unconscious and therefore lacks capacity.
- Discuss with the next of kin/family if the patient has a legally valid advanced directive about refusing a transfusion. It is important that this specifically mentions that a refusal of treatment is valid even if there is a threat to life. Patients may carry an advance directive card on their person.
- If they do not, then ask if there is a lasting power of attorney (LPA) and if so, are they specifically an LPA for health. Remember that for an LPA to refuse life-saving treatment for a patient it must be very clearly stated on the LPA that they can do this.
- Confirm if the patient would accept other blood products or would accept autotransfusion.

Patient Safety
- If there are no advanced directives and the patient is unable to consent then a best interest decision must be taken in an emergency. It appears likely the patient will need a blood transfusion or they will die.
- One of the principles of a best interest decision is that your interventions should be the least restrictive of their future options. Clearly, avoiding death is the least restrictive option.

Initiative
- You can outline initial mechanisms that may delay the need for transfusion, such as checking whether they have a cell salvage machine available or have prepared blood

for auto-transfusion. N.B. this usually will not be available in time to help in an emergency like this.
- Assign a member of staff, preferably a senior nurse to go and calmly discuss with the family member away from the resuscitation bay.
- You may assign a member of staff to call the Jehovah's Watchtower service for advice. However, this should not delay treatment, as this is a best interest decision.

Escalate
- Communicate the issue to the trauma team lead clearly and succinctly.
- Escalate this case to the responsible consultant.
- Escalate to the legal department as soon as it is safe to do so.

Support
- The patient: ensure the trauma call continues to be run in the best interests of the patient until they are stabilised. If this requires blood transfusion to prevent serious harm or death, then in the absence of legally valid documentation of a refusal to accept blood products, then blood products should be used if there are no other options.
- Yourself: a trauma call like this, coupled with the added complication of the blood transfusion issue, would be extremely stressful. Ensure you have time after the patient is stabilised to have a break, discuss with a senior such as your CS/ES.
- Your team: ensure you debrief after the case so that decisions can be assessed, and the team can be supported.
- The family: they may be very upset at the decision and having a regular named point of contact to discuss with them would be helpful.

Document/Reflect
- Ensure all conversations are fully and clearly documented, and the reasons for the decisions are clearly stated.
- These are relatively complicated topics and a refresher teaching session on consent, capacity, and the refusal of life-saving treatment may be helpful for your department.
- Reflect in your ePortfolio on this acutely stressful scenario.

The family member finds a letter from the patient in which he mentions that it is against his religious beliefs to have a transfusion, and he wouldn't want to have one. They say this means you can't give him a transfusion. How do you proceed?
You would check if this was a valid legally binding advanced directive, and whether it specifically mentions that this is the case even if the alternative is death. Otherwise, in this emergency scenario this paper does not change your decision to transfuse.

The family member becomes verbally aggressive and shouts profanities at you at the edge of the resus bay. You are concerned they may escalate to using physical aggression. How would you manage this situation?
The approach to an aggressive patient is highlighted in Scenario 7.7 and a similar approach should be used for a family member. We would add that in this specific

scenario you would need to use your judgement to factor in the added pressure on the relative due to the immensely high stress of the situation and how this may be affecting their behaviour. Regardless, abusive behaviour should not be tolerated.

7.17 Research Fraud

You are an orthopaedic CT2 involved in collecting long-term follow-up data for publication comparing patient outcomes following different operative approaches to a fractured NOF. You send the excel spreadsheet of your findings to your registrar, who returns it with some of the raw data edited to produce a more impressive result. How do you proceed?

Issues

- Research ethics, integrity, and professionalism: tampering with data is clearly in breach of fundamental principles of research ethics.
- Patient safety: possible dissemination of incorrect data which can affect patient care in the future.

Seek Information

- Discuss with your registrar what you have noticed. Explore if there are any explanations you are missing – for example, the registrar has access to data which you do not have. If you have concerns, it would be important for you to review this data yourself. Check previous data you have worked on together to see if there have also been discrepancies.

Patient Safety

- Although not directly affected, it is worth thinking about possible long-term effects from incorrect data being disseminated, such as the adoption by other surgeons of a less favourable operative technique based on the findings.

Initiative

- Raise this directly with your registrar in the first instance, explain why this is unacceptable and you are not happy to proceed with the project in this manner. If there are concerns about the integrity of the research and the data has been submitted to any conferences or journals, you should withdraw the work pending resolution of this situation.

Escalate

- If you are concerned that they are purposefully editing data, then explain that you need to escalate this to a senior. If there is a consultant in charge of the project, this is the obvious person, but your CS/ES would also be reasonable. The head of department would be the next person to contact.
- If you have concerns that the issue is not being adequately resolved locally, this should be escalated as per the local research ethics policy. Confidential support can be found from the research services department or a subcommittee of the research ethics committee.

- This behaviour raises the possibility that the registrar has done this before – this would need investigating. It is not your place to be investigating this yourself.

Support
- The research team: by helping in any investigations going forward.

Document/Reflect
- It is worth writing a contemporaneous account of what happened both for the purposes of reflection and to ensure if this is investigated further you have clear documentation of the incident.

The registrar is angry with your response, and the next time you are in theatre together, it becomes clear that he will not facilitate your learning – what do you do?
Recognise that this would be a difficult scenario to be encountered with, but that you have done nothing wrong – you have acted with integrity during this process. In the first instance it is worth discussing this directly with your registrar to see if you can 'clear the air' together. If this is not the case, or you feel unable to broach this, then it is important to escalate this to your CS/ES. In the interim, discuss with the rota coordinator about being put on different lists to the registrar, something which is usually easily facilitated. It is important to resolve this as (1) this form of unprofessional and rude behaviour is known to result in worse patient outcomes (2) it is limiting your training opportunities and (3) this form of behaviour must be challenged to protect future trainees from being exposed to it.

7.18 Inadequate Training Opportunities
You are an orthopaedic CT1, you have been on the ward for two months with almost no theatre or clinic time. The service is extremely busy, and you are often short-staffed. You feel you are not progressing in training. Today is a rare day that you are scheduled to go to theatre but have been told by the on-call registrar to remain on the ward as it is busy.

Issues
- Patient safety: in the short term you must ensure there is sufficient cover to keep patients safe on the ward. However, going forward there may be safety concerns if the department is regularly understaffed.
- Personal development and training: if you are not getting adequate surgical training then this must be escalated. Core surgical training places a lot of demands on a trainee, but these demands must be balanced with also getting adequate theatre exposure.

Seek Information
- Is there anything specific that is making the wards too busy for you to go to theatre (e.g. an acutely unwell patient that needs urgent review)? Are there jobs that could be completed quickly to allow you to go to theatre later that morning?
- Determine staffing levels across the department for the day.

Patient Safety

- If there is no cover, or there is short staffing, you must look after the ward patients. Your training opportunities are a longer-term issue.

Initiative

- This case is about demonstrating proactivity when facing a common problem in core surgical training – the need to balance service provision with theatre time and how you make plans over the short and long term.
- For this day specifically, see if there are other juniors who may be more suitable to cover the ward who have had more theatre exposure recently, discussing this with the registrar on call, the rota coordinator, and your junior doctor colleagues.
- To address this issue going forward, begin by looking at the rota and ensuring it matches your job plan and determine how much theatre time is on there. Compare this to the JCST (Joint Committee on Surgical Training) recommendations. Ensure the burden of ward cover and on-call cover is being split fairly and evenly amongst the junior doctors. See how many days you were scheduled for theatre/clinic and how many times you have been unable to go due to the ward commitments. Discuss with your colleagues to see if they have had a similar experience in the department. Amalgamating the experience of multiple trainees across multiple weeks will make trends stronger. Speaking to previous trainees can help you to see if this issue is generalisable to the department and may also give you advice on strategies to mitigate the issue.
- In the meantime, ensure you are taking full advantage of the opportunities that are available to you – for example that you are doing procedures while on call, reading up around interesting ward cases that you see, and teaching medical students. Ensure other aspects of your surgical training are being worked on in the interim – anatomy, courses, publications, audits, and membership examinations can be prioritised in the short term.

Escalate

- You should escalate first to your CS/ES; they can help you uncover whether there is anything you could change about your own approach. You can then discuss any systemic issues you have highlighted such as a lack of staffing. They can also advocate for you to get more training opportunities and help amend the rota or even start the process of hiring more staff if required. You may be able to come up with a plan where you have protected days blocked off for theatre in advance. Remember that your ES/CS are there to help you – the discussion should be open and proactive, not confrontational.
- If this fails to help, then given this is a training issue, escalating to your TPD would be appropriate. In extreme cases it may be that the rotation is not sufficiently resourced to be a training rotation. Some regions also have surgical tutors or regional representatives that you can speak to before escalation to the TPD.

Support

- Yourself: ensure you are adequately supported by supervisors, colleagues and friends as you try to advocate for yourself in a trying situation.

- Your team: be flexible in covering shifts while the rota is changed. Be realistic in understanding that staffing issues will take time to change – do not lose heart and look after yourself in the meantime.

Document/Reflect

- Ensure your portfolio is fully up to date, that you have reflected on the issue and that you have clearly mapped which opportunities you need to achieve your objectives.

Tell me about a time where you have struggled to get training opportunities and how did you react

Follow-up questions could relate to your own experience, and it is helpful to have two to three rehearsed examples of situations you have faced that map to multiple themes that may be asked about, such as taking initiative, advocating for yourself in the face of challenges, and taking responsibility for your own learning. There are typically only one to two minutes for these questions, so it is quite difficult to recall and clearly articulate a succinct story on the spot without having already prepared it.

A good answer should acknowledge the current issues with service provision in training jobs, while highlighting concrete examples of times you have improved your training output. For example, perhaps you have drawn up a plan with your supervisor to get you into theatre more, asked to be with a specific senior on multiple occasions to build training rapport, used a busy placement in a prestigious unit to pursue research, or run a bedside teaching program for medical students on a job where you are on the ward a lot. Almost anything can be construed as a training opportunity; what is important is that you demonstrate your proactivity in the face of adversity.

7.19 Consent for a Child

You are the plastic surgery CT1. You have been referred a 15-year-old boy who has an abscess in the first webspace of his hand, with an area of spreading cellulitis around it. Given its size and location, formal washout will need to occur under GA. When you broach this with the parents, they are adamant that they will not allow their child to have a GA. They would like to try homeopathic or other alternative medicine in the first instance.

Issues

- Patient safety: you have identified that there is an acute infection that needs source control.
- Consent and capacity in a child.

Seek Information

- Make sure you are confident in the diagnosis and management plan you have for this patient; getting early senior input if you are unsure would be appropriate, particularly as this decision rests in large part on whether a general anaesthetic is required or not.
- Explore with the parents what their concerns are regarding a general anaesthetic. See if there are worries or preconceptions that they have about this. Explore what the other treatment options they have been reading about entail. Ensure this

conversation happens in private, away from your bleep if possible, and is in a non-confrontational and non-judgemental manner. As the case progresses it will be essential the parents feel listened to, and their views are respected.
- During the conversation ask for the patient's input; you can use this to begin to determine the ability of the patient to consent for themselves

Patient Safety
- The child's safety is paramount. Ensure they remain clinically stable during this discussion.
- It is important this scenario is managed carefully – damaging the parents' trust in the medical profession may result in the family not seeking help in the future.

Initiative
- Ensure you have a strong grasp of the condition and the case in question, with access to relevant history and investigations, so you can have a proper discussion with the parents. It is important you explain the possible outcomes if the child does not have surgery. Assess if there is any possibility for the procedure to safely occur under a local or regional block.
- Assess the patient's capacity to make their own decision. This would be in line with the principles of Gillick competence. It may be that the child can consent for themselves. Note that overriding the parents' wishes is a serious situation that will need to be handled carefully; it can cause a breakdown of trust, prevent them seeking medical care in the future, and may make postoperative care (where the parents will likely be needed) more difficult.

Escalation
- It would be important to get your senior involved in this case. If nothing else, the family may feel more comfortable after speaking to someone more senior.
- Offer for the family to speak to the anaesthetics team (as their concerns appear to be related to the GA).
- In extremis, you may require advice from your hospital's legal department. This would be after it had already been escalated to your seniors, and in only a small subset of circumstances would it be necessary.

Support
- Support your team: ensure everything else is ready, for example bloods are taken, consent form is prepped.
- Support the patient: ensure they remain stable and help the situation towards resolution. Begin non-operative management with antibiotics and fluids as required.
- Support the family: this will be a highly stressful time for the parents as well. Remember, they will almost certainly believe they have the best interests of their child at heart as well!

Document/Reflect
- Whatever the outcome, it is essential that you meticulously document the discussion that was had. Ensure the correct consent form is used.

– This may have been a stressful situation to find yourself in, and reflecting on it with your supervisor would be useful. Take the initiative by reading up on the law regarding children and consenting; it would make a useful departmental refresher.

After assessing the child, you feel they do not have capacity. The parents are still refusing to proceed with treatment; what do you do?

Ensure your senior is involved if not already – this will need escalation to the consultant on call. Ensure there is nothing you can do to help the child gain capacity (are they in pain or dehydrated which is distracting them?); your senior should also assess them to confirm this. Once all avenues with the parents have been exhausted, you would need to make a decision in the patient's best interest. This would be escalated through your seniors, the hospital legal team, your defence union, and the courts as appropriate. In an emergency, life-saving treatment should be given, and legal sanction for this can be sought as soon as possible afterwards.

The child has capacity but is refusing treatment; how do you proceed?

You would need to fully assess their capacity, get a second opinion, and fully explore their ideas and concerns, any preconceptions they have, or other treatments they had in mind. The legal situation around a competent child who refuses treatment is complex, and this scenario should be quickly escalated up, and legal advice should be sought. The Court of Protection can overrule a competent child's decision in some instances, but these unusual instances are taken on a case-by-case basis.

You have gone off shift. The parents feel that their child is deteriorating, and do not feel the clinical team are taking these concerns seriously? Do the parents have a right to a second opinion?

As of April 2024, the NHS is rolling out a new patient safety initiative through 'Martha's Rule'. This will allow patients and families to request a review from a critical care outreach team 24/7 if they have concerns about their clinical condition. This follows the tragic death of 13-year-old Martha Mills, whose care was not escalated to ICU despite her family's concerns about her deteriorating condition.

From where did the idea of Gillick competence arise?

A case was brought by Victoria Gillick against her local authority in the 1980s arguing that her daughters should not have access to contraceptive support without her consent. It was eventually escalated to the High Court, where it was ruled that a child can be assessed for competence in the same way as an adult, and if the child is competent, parents do not necessarily have a parental right to intervene. This applies for children under the age of 16 – children who are 16 and 17 are assumed to have capacity in the UK.

8 Introduction to the Clinical Stations

8.1 Overview of the Clinical Stations

The CST interviews include two five-minute clinical stations. Clinical stations can broadly be split into:

– Patients presenting in trauma scenarios requiring a trauma A–E approach.
– Patients presenting acutely unwell with surgical pathologies, usually on the ward or in the emergency department, who require an acute A–E workup.
– Stable patients, usually presenting in outpatient settings. While a brief A–E assessment is required to ensure the patient is stable, a greater onus should be placed on subsequent history, investigations, and management. Outpatient scenarios appear to be far less common than acutely unwell or trauma patients.

8.2 The Template A–E Approach

The importance of a strong A–E approach during your CST interview cannot be over-stated. It should form the starting point for every clinical scenario. It provides a structure for you to build more advanced knowledge into your answers. It shows examiners that you are going to be a safe and competent core surgical trainee. Recognising unwell patients, beginning to stabilise them, and escalating to your seniors is what is expected primarily of a core trainee. Once you have demonstrated this to the examiners, you can show off the more advanced knowledge that will put you ahead of the pack.

We would advise the following steps to prepare for the clinical scenarios:

1. Write a structure for a generic A–E assessment for both acutely unwell cases and trauma cases. Important resources for you to consolidate include CCRISP (Care of the Critically Ill Surgical Patient), ALS (Advanced Life Support), and ATLS (Advanced Trauma Life Support). Naturally you will need to condense your approach down – reading off the entire ATLS A–E would take far too long. Ensure you remain reasonably comprehensive in your approach – leave the examiners in no doubt that you can perform a thorough A–E.

2. Practise bringing your total speech down to around the two-to-three-minute mark. This may seem difficult to begin with, but with repetition and small adjustments to your script, you can produce a succinct but comprehensive approach which offers sufficient time to answer follow-up questions.

3. Once you have this A–E 'scaffold', work on adjusting your approach to a given scenario. This might include expanding a specific component of the assessment that you know is relevant to the case at hand or referencing important differentials during your workup. The ability to adapt an A–E assessment to a given scenario will mark

you out as a candidate who can both understand the scenario from a clinical point of view and can think on their feet.

4. Once you are confident in your adapted A–E, practise follow-up questions that could be asked for each scenario. A comprehensive, tailored A–E will likely have answered many of the questions the examiners have for you. Remember that producing a comprehensive A–E must take priority over preparing niche follow-up questions which may or may not come up!

Example A–E Approach (Shortform) for the Acutely Unwell Surgical Patient

Introduction

Airway: ensure patent and unobstructed.

Breathing: RR, O_2 sats, commence 15 L O_2, examine chest +/− adjuncts (e.g. ABG, CXR).

Circulation: BP, HR, central and peripheral pulses + CRT, IV access, bloods +/− fluids +/− catheter +/− electrocardiography (ECG).

Disability: AVPU score, pupillary examination, capillary blood glucose (CBG), temperature.

Exposure: perform a full focused [system] examination including [specifics relevant to case], maintaining patient temperature and dignity.

AAPS

– Analgesia.
– Antiemetics.
– +/− Pregnancy test.
– Senior discussion.

AAPS

AAPS is a simple mnemonic to remember four things to quickly reel off after your A–E which you might be inclined to forget about in the heat of the moment. Most patients will benefit from analgesia/antiemetics, all women of childbearing age must have a pregnancy test, and all patients will need some kind of discussion with your senior.

History, Notes, Investigations

– History: full focused clinical history using the allergies, medications, past medical history, last meal, events (AMPLE) structure.
– Notes: examine patient's notes/op notes/ward round entries/drug chart as relevant.
– Investigations: arrange further investigations as required.

AMPLE History

An 'AMPLE history' is a useful aid-memoir for the emergency surgical history, which stands for Allergies, Medications, Past medical history, Last meal/oral intake, and Events leading to presentation.

Additional Notes

- You should be going back and re-assessing the patient from 'A' after each intervention to determine if it has had an effect.
- If life-threatening pathology has been identified in your A–E you should manage this before moving on.
- In cases of potential sepsis, you should be initiating SEPSIS 6: take blood cultures, lactate, and monitor urine output; give O_2, antibiotics, and fluids. All of these steps can be completed by the end of your initial workup.

Example A–E Approach (Longform) for the Acutely Unwell Surgical Patient

I would immediately assess the patient using a CCRISP-guided A–E approach. I would first ensure the airway was patent, and that the patient could protect their airway. I would then get an up-to-date respiratory rate and oxygen saturations, start 15 L oxygen through a non-rebreather mask, and then inspect, palpate, percuss, and auscultate the chest. If there were signs of respiratory distress, I would consider adjuncts such as an ABG and chest X-ray.

If stable, I would get an updated blood pressure and heart rate, examine the central and peripheral capillary refill times and pulses, and get IV access with a large bore cannula in each ACF. At this point I would take off a full set of bloods including [ ].

I would consider starting a fluid bolus at this point with [ ]ml warmed IV crystalloid. I would consider catheterising the patient and getting an ECG.

If I was happy with my assessment so far, I would briefly examine the patient's neurological system with an AVPU score and pupillary examination, and also get a CBG and a temperature.

I would go back and repeat my assessments to assess the response to any interventions I have initiated, and, if happy, perform a full focused [ ] exam including [ ].

At this point, I would offer analgesia, antiemetics, (a pregnancy test), and alert my senior.

Finally, I would obtain a focused clinical history using the AMPLE structure, examine the patient's notes, and arrange further investigations as required.

This is a rough template for your approach. Once you master this basic blueprint you will need to tailor it to the scenario at hand. Occasionally the scenario will not start at the bedside, but with a phone call or bleep. Start your workup on the phone to demonstrate that you have paid attention to the vignette and are being practical and efficient in your approach. For example, when informed by phone about an unwell postoperative patient:

This patient sounds acutely unwell, and I would go and assess them immediately. Over the phone, I would ask the nursing staff to take a new set of observations, prepare a kit for IV access and have the patient notes at the bedside. I would let my senior know I was going to review the patient. Once at the bedside . . . .

Let's imagine you have been given the following clinical scenario:

You are the on-call general surgical senior house officer (SHO). You are called by a nurse on the ward asking you to review a 59-year-old male complaining of severe abdominal pain. He is febrile at 38.4°C, his BP is 95/60 and his HR is 110. The patient is five days post resection of low rectal cancer with primary anastomosis.

In your head, you should already have an idea of the top differentials in this scenario (anastomotic leak/intra-abdominal collection or abscess), and your A–E should be moderated to demonstrate this. For example:

This patient sounds acutely unwell, is shocked, and given the clinical vignette, I am particularly concerned about possible anastomotic leak or postoperative intra-abdominal collection or abscess. I would go and assess them immediately using a CCRISP guided A–E approach. On the phone I would ask the nursing staff to take a set of observations and prepare the patient's notes, and I would let my senior know I was going to review the patient.

I would first ensure the airway was patent, and that the patient could protect their airway. I would then get an up-to-date respiratory rate and oxygen sats, start 15 L oxygen through a non-rebreather mask, and then inspect, palpate, percuss, and auscultate the chest. If there were signs of respiratory distress, such as from abdominal pain splinting the diaphragm, I would consider adjuncts such as an ABG and CXR.

If this is stable, I would get an updated blood pressure and heart rate, examine the central and peripheral capillary refill times and pulses, and get good IV access with a large bore cannula in each ACF. At this point, I would take a full set of bloods including full blood count (FBC), U&Es, LFTs, as well as group and saves with a mind to potential operative management, a VBG to get a quick assessment of their Hb and lactate, and blood cultures. I would start a fluid bolus at this point with 20 ml/kg warmed crystalloid as per CCRSIP guidelines for hypotensive patients. I would catheterise the patient to monitor urine output and get an ECG. Further fluid would be titrated to response.

While the patient is being fluid resuscitated, I would perform a brief neurological examination with an AVPU score and a pupillary examination. I would get a CBG, and a temperature.

I would go back and repeat my assessments, and if happy, perform a full focused abdominal exam, including examining the wound sites, and looking particularly for signs of peritonism which may be caused by an anastomotic leak.

At this point, I would offer analgesia and antiemetics, and alert my senior. I would examine the patient's operation notes, ward round entries since the operation, drug chart, recent investigations, and the trend in their observations. I would take a focused clinical history with an AMPLE structure before ordering further investigations as appropriate. Given my concerns about possible intra-abdominal sepsis, I would ensure empirical antibiotics are given urgently, completing the SEPSIS 6 protocol.

This answer is structured, comprehensive, adapted to the patient at hand, completes the SEPSIS 6 protocol, and demonstrates you have a differential in mind. It is succinct and can be read at a comfortable pace in less than two and a half minutes. It also sets you up nicely for follow-up questions about further investigations and management. These will be discussed in more depth later in the book.

Example A–E Approach (Shortform) for Trauma Scenarios

Introduction: ensure patient is seen in suitable area (move to resus if required).

C-spine: ensure triple immobilised until cleared.

Airway: ensure patent.

Breathing: RR, O$_2$ sats, commence 15 L O$_2$, examine chest wall +/− adjuncts (e.g. ABG, CXR).

Circulation: BP, HR, central and peripheral pulses + CRT, IV access, bloods +/− fluids/blood products +/− catheter +/− ECG +/− splints/binders.

Disability: GCS + pupillary examination, CBG, temperature.

Exposure: expose pt, logroll and full top-to-toe assessment (to identify life-threatening pathology), focused examination of [ ], including [ ], maintaining patient temperature and dignity.

Extra Steps (AAPS)

- Analgesia.
- Antiemetics.
- +/− Pregnancy test.
- Senior discussion.

History, Notes, Investigations

- History: full focused clinical history using the AMPLE structure.
- Notes: examine patient's notes.
- Investigations: arrange further investigations as required.

N.B. in a formal ATLS A–E assessment, during 'exposure' you are advised to perform a logroll and top-to-toe assessment to identify any life-threatening pathology you may have missed. This is followed by a more comprehensive top-to-toe evaluation (starting from the scalp) to identify any other concomitant injuries as part of a secondary survey. Given the comprehensive nature of this latter evaluation, it is unlikely you would need to describe this in detail during a five-minute trauma scenario.

Not all post-trauma scenarios will require a full ATLS A–E. If a stable patient is referred by the emergency department for a specialty review following trauma, it is likely they will have had a primary and secondary survey performed already if this was required. However, the safest approach is to assume these have not occurred. If it is specified that they have, a brief A–E to reassess them and ensure nothing was missed would suffice, and more time can then be spent on investigations, management, and follow-up questions.

Example A–E Approach (Longform) for ATLS Scenarios

On my way to review the patient, I would ensure a trauma call had been put out, and that my senior was aware of the situation. I would receive an SBAR handover before assessing the patient using an ATLS A–E approach.

I would begin by triple immobilising the patient's C-spine using collar, blocks and tape. I would check for a patent, unobstructed airway that the patient is able to protect.

Next, I would assess for signs of life-threatening chest pathology using an inspect, palpate, percuss, auscultate approach. I would get an up-to-date respiratory rate and oxygen saturations. I would give the patient 15 L oxygen through a non rebreather mask. I'd request adjuncts including ABG and portable chest X-ray as required.

If satisfied with breathing, I would assess for signs of haemodynamic instability by getting an up-to-date blood pressure and heart rate, assessing central and peripheral capillary refill times and pulses, and assessing the warmth and colour of the patient's extremities. I would ensure I had good IV access with a wide bore cannula in each ACF, and while these were being inserted, I would ensure a full set of bloods including group and save/cross match, clotting, VBG and [ ] were taken.

I would assess for signs of haemorrhage, performing adjunct investigations as required. I would give 1 L warmed IV crystalloid fluid as per ATLS guidelines, with additional fluids titrated to response. I would consider putting out a major haemorrhage call. I would consider a pelvic binder if there are concerns about pelvic injury and catheterise the patient if there were no concerns about urethral injury. I would also listen to the heart sounds and perform an ECG.

After reassessing the response to my current interventions, I would check the patient's temperature and CBG and assess their GCS and pupillary responses. I would then expose the patient, being mindful of the risk of hypothermia and preserving their dignity, whilst I conducted a head-to-toe examination, including a log roll, to ensure no life-threatening injuries had been missed. I would ensure they had analgesia and antiemetics prescribed, a pregnancy test had been performed, and my senior had been informed. I would take a full history using the AMPLE structure, perform a comprehensive top-to-toe examination to identify any other concomitant pathology as part of a secondary survey. Given the history, I would ensure I had performed a focused examination of [ ], looking for [ ]. I would then order further investigations such as [ ].

Clearly this is a very broad approach. Let's imagine you are given this scenario:

You are the on-call general surgical SHO and are called to resus to assess a patient with breathing difficulties after being stabbed in the right side of the chest. RR 28, saturations 88% on room air.

In this situation, you should be expanding the 'breathing' section of your assessment to provide more detail on the life-threatening chest pathologies you are concerned about (in this instance key differentials for right-sided penetrating chest trauma are tension pneumothorax, open pneumothorax, and haemothorax). Once you have covered your introduction, C-spine, and airway...

...Next, I would ensure the trachea was central, examine the neck veins, look for signs of respiratory distress, and then inspect, palpate, percuss, and auscultate the chest wall, looking for equal chest expansion and any signs of chest trauma or open wounds. I would get an up-to-date respiratory rate and oxygen saturations. I would give the patient 15 L oxygen through a non-rebreather mask. Given there are concerns about respiratory distress, I would ensure a portable chest X-ray and ABG were performed, although this should not delay decompression and definitive management of a tension pneumothorax if the clinical picture is in keeping with this...

You have now made it clear that you are correctly focusing on life-threatening chest pathology and have an idea how to manage them. At this point, the examiners will either stop you and ask you to expand on 'breathing' further (e.g. by asking 'what are your differentials' or by volunteering information picked up on your examination), or they will say nothing. In which case, to finish your breathing section and move on you can say...

...I would reassess the patient's breathing after my interventions. If they have now stabilised, I would move on to assess their circulation...

You can see how adapting the structure of your A–E allows you to signpost that you know what is going on and start to answer follow-up questions in your initial assessment.

Let's imagine a second trauma scenario:

You are the on-call general surgical SHO. You are called to resus to assess a shocked male who has been involved in a road traffic accident. They are complaining of left-sided abdominal pain. Obs: RR 20 sats 98% RA, BP 100/60 HR 120.

In this situation you should be tailoring your A–E to put extra onus on 'circulation', while still ensuring you do not miss anything in the assessment. Once you have covered C-spine, airway, and breathing, your approach may be...

...Once satisfied with breathing, I would get an up-to-date blood pressure and heart rate, assess the central and peripheral capillary refill times and pulses, and assess the warmth and colour of the patient's extremities. I would ensure I had IV access with a wide bore cannula in each ACF and that a full set of bloods were taken including group and save/cross match, VBG (for a rapid assessment of their haemoglobin and lactate), and clotting (given possible haemorrhage), as well as baseline FBC and U&Es with a mind to potential operative management.

I would begin with a bolus 1 L of warmed IV crystalloid and assess the response. Hypotension in the trauma setting should be considered haemorrhage until proven otherwise. As such, I would assess for potential sources of lethal haemorrhage (thorax, abdomen, pelvis, long bones, and external bleeding) and consider adjuvant investigations for this. In this situation, a FAST scan would be appropriate if there are concerns about intra-abdominal haemorrhage. I would put out a major haemorrhage call as early replacement with blood products is required. If there were concerns about pelvic injury, I would place a pelvic binder on the patient. If there are no concerns about urethral injury, I would catheterise the patient. I would also listen to the heart sounds and ask for an ECG to be performed...

In this situation, you have confidently started the investigation and management of intra-abdominal haemorrhage, without 'nailing your colours to the mast' of one specific diagnosis, such as splenic rupture, which it would be premature to do here without further information. Again, examiners may stop you and ask you further questions about abdominal trauma or allow you to finish your assessment.

8.3 Final Remarks

Be prepared for the trauma A–E to take longer than the acutely unwell A–E; this was our experience. Your trauma assessment should still aim to come in under three minutes for a given scenario.

We would strongly recommend that you become confident in approaching common postoperative scenarios. You should have clear differentials in mind for postoperative shortness of breath/hypoxia, postoperative fever, and postoperative fall in urine output. These are covered in the scenarios which follow.

Avoid memorising the scripts above word for word. Instead, you should be reading the resources we described above (namely ATLS and CCRISP resources), and should therefore have the depth of understanding to generate your own script. This will allow you to add your own touches which feel natural for you and the way you speak – small changes can make your A–E stand out. For example, adding in that you would take the time to explain what is going on to a patient after your trauma workup shows you are thinking holistically about a patient going through an extremely difficult process.

The cases that we have showcased in this book use a combination of verbatim answers *in italics*, and bullet-point answers. The verbatim answers will allow you to get an understanding of the flow of an entire complete answer, while the bullet points provide you with the scope to flesh out more complete answers of your own. In earlier cases, the A–E assessments tend to be written verbatim, but there are verbatim answers to follow-up questions written sporadically throughout the cases. Note that as answers become bullet points, basic aspects of the A–E assessment are excluded from the model answer. It is expected these will still be included in your workup, but the A–E notes will instead cover areas more pertinent to the case at hand. A range of follow up questions have been included, some of which are designed to really stretch candidates and may be beyond what is expected as a CT1. However, they contain clinically relevant information that helps you understand a topic in more depth, and therefore stand out at interview. Remember that a strong initial workup is by far the most important part of each scenario.

Clinical Scenarios

9.1 Lower Limb Trauma

You are the orthopaedic CT1 on call and are called to assess a 23-year-old male who is in majors after being knocked off his motorbike by a car while travelling at 40 mph. He has marked swelling of his right and left thighs which appear deformed. There are no skin breakages and there are no other obvious injuries. His observations are HR 110, BP 100/40, RR 16, Sats 98% on RA, apyrexial.

Before you begin: This is a haemodynamically unstable patient following high-energy trauma; they should be managed in resus. They are in class II–III shock. Ensure a trauma call has been put out, your senior is aware, and immediately go to see the patient. Do not overlook the possibility that there is another source of bleeding, and that there is a pelvic fracture alongside this severe femoral injury.

This patient has suffered a high-energy trauma and is in class II–III shock. A trauma call should be put out, the patient should be moved to resus immediately, and the patient should be assessed using an ATLS A–E approach. I would alert my senior while on the way down to review them as it is highly likely I will need urgent senior support.

A–E
C-Spine

Given the mechanism of injury, I would ensure the C-spine is triple immobilised with collar, blocks and tape, pending clearance of the C-spine.

Airway

I would ensure the patient has a patent, unobstructed airway.

Breathing

I would assess for life-threatening respiratory pathology using an inspect, palpate, percuss, and auscultate approach. I would get an up-to-date RR and O_2 sats and give the patient 15 L oxygen through a non-rebreather mask. I'd request adjuncts including ABG and portable chest X-ray as required.

Circulation

Haemodynamic instability in a trauma patient is due to haemorrhage until proven otherwise. I would check for signs of external haemorrhage, as well as assessing the chest, abdomen, pelvis, and long bones for signs of bleeding. If there were any concerns about pelvic injury I would place a pelvic binder, which should be centred at the level of the greater trochanters. Given the patient is unstable, a bedside eFAST scan would be a useful adjunct to assess for sources of bleeding. I would ensure that wide bore IV access is obtained in each ACF and a full set of bloods, including a VBG, clotting, and group and saves (to cross match four units initially) are sent. I would start a 1 L warmed IV crystalloid fluid bolus and assess their response. I would consider giving IV tranexamic acid. If I was concerned about haemorrhage, I would place a major haemorrhage call and begin resuscitating with blood products as early as possible. A catheter should be placed to monitor urine output.

The assessment has already highlighted possible sources of bleeding in the thighs bilaterally. The deformity of the legs makes me concerned for femoral shaft fractures. Traction and splinting of the affected limbs will help reduce the fracture which in turn will help control both pain and bleeding. Neurovascular assessments should be performed both pre and post fracture manipulation. Ongoing bleeding or concerns about the neurovascular status of the legs would necessitate proceeding urgently to CEPOD, and if so, starting theatre workup at this point is necessary. Torniquets can be used to compress both arterial and venous flow to the limb in the short term, with a named individual responsible for calling out every 15 minutes that the torniquet is on.

Disability

I would ensure the patient's GCS is monitored and ensure they do not become hypothermic given the haemorrhage. I would document the pupillary size and reactivity, the presence of lateralising neurological signs and, if present, determine the level of spinal cord injury.

Exposure

A full top-to-toe examination including a log roll to identify other life-threatening injuries should be performed. I would take a 'look, feel, move approach' to examine the affected limbs, ensuring that neurovascular status was documented.

AAPS

I would ensure the patient had adequate analgesia. I would inform my senior of my examination findings and ask them to urgently review the patient.

History, Notes, Investigations

If able, I would take an AMPLE history from the patient. I would be sure to check for any previous bleeding disorders. If they are now stable enough to proceed to radiology, I would request a trauma CT, ensuring that the thighs and shins are both included (or that XRs of these areas are ordered) to check for more distal injury.

- N.B. CT trauma series typically only contains CT head, spine, thorax, abdo, and pelvis unless specified. Otherwise, XRs should be ordered for other affected areas.

Preliminary and Further Management

Following resuscitation and initial fracture manipulation this patient will likely need to go to theatre for fracture stabilisation. In unstable trauma patients, temporary stabilisation with external fixation should be considered, with a plan for definitive fixation in the coming days when the patient is more stable. I would speak to the theatre coordinator, anaesthetist on call, and my senior. Given the severity of his clinical state he may require ITU postoperatively, so I would speak to the ITU registrar on call. I would ensure he had all relevant preoperative workup, was made nil by mouth, consented by someone appropriate to do so, and marked. I would ensure ongoing resuscitation was taking place while this was happening. Long bone fractures can lead to compartment syndrome and so this patient will need close monitoring perioperatively.

What are the types of shock? How can these be clinically differentiated?
- **Hypovolaemic**: hypotension, tachycardia, peripherally shut down. Typically haemorrhage-related in trauma scenarios.
- **Cardiogenic**: hypotension, tachycardia, signs of peripheral/central fluid overload. In trauma look for high-energy trauma to the chest.
- **Anaphylactic**: hypotension, tachycardia, urticaria, dyspnoea.
- **Septic**: hypotension, tachycardia, pink/warm/flushed skin.
- **Neurogenic**: hypotension, bradycardia, widespread peripheral dilatation. Caused by neurological injury causing inhibition of sympathetic drive or increased parasympathetic drive. N.B. neurogenic shock and spinal shock are not the same but are often incorrectly used interchangeably.

What are the complications of a massive blood transfusion?
Complications can be categorised into volume related, homeostasis disruption, and immune system dysfunction.
- **Volume related**: transfusion-associated cardiac overload (TACO).
- **Homeostasis disruption**: electrolyte abnormalities, for example hyperkalaemia (from red cell lysis) and hypocalcaemia (from blood products containing citrate, which chelates calcium); coagulopathy caused by imbalance of clotting factors; hypothermia.
- **Immune system dysfunction**: transfusion-associated lung injury (TRALI).

What is the trauma triad of death?
Hypothermia, coagulopathy, and acidosis. These three factors interact to cause a positive feedback loop: bleeding diminishes oxygen delivery (causing acidosis via anaerobic respiration) and loss of body heat (causing hypothermia). These then in turn slow the coagulation cascade, reducing clotting and therefore worsening bleeding.

9.2 Spreading Skin Changes
You are the CT1 on call overnight for orthopaedics at a district general hospital. You are called by ITU to assess a 67-year-old diabetic man who has been intubated having been critically unwell following a severe bout of *E. coli* gastroenteritis. They are concerned about a new dark, blistering rash on the patient's right thigh which is spreading. How do you proceed?

Before you begin: The most important differential to consider is necrotising fasciitis. This is a life-threatening emergency (mortality roughly 25%) in which infection spreads rapidly along fascial planes. This condition should be mentioned as part of your differential in your opening sentence.

This patient is acutely unwell, and the presence of a new progressing rash, in the presence of risk factors, makes me particularly concerned about the possibility of necrotising fasciitis. Other differentials would include cellulitis and drug reactions. This is a life-threatening emergency that must be assessed immediately using a CCRISP-guided A-to-E approach.

A–E

Airway

The patient is currently intubated so their airway should be protected.

Breathing

I would start 15 L of oxygen via a non-rebreather mask and get an up-to-date respiratory rate and oxygen saturations before assessing the chest with an inspect, palpate, auscultate, and percuss approach. I would consider the use of an ABG or chest X-ray as an adjunct if any respiratory pathology was identified. I would start high-flow oxygen.

Circulation

Once satisfied with their breathing, I would ask for an up-to-date blood pressure and heart rate, obtain IV access with a large bore cannula in each ACF, and take a full blood panel including VBG, FBC and U&Es, blood cultures, clotting, and group and saves. I would give the patient bolus IV fluids titrated to response, commence broad spectrum antibiotics, and catheterise to monitor urine output, thus completing the SEPSIS 6 protocol.

Disability

I would perform a rapid neurological evaluation with a GCS and pupillary examination, as well as getting their temperature and a CBG.

Exposure

I would then perform a focused examination of the rash, as well as a full top-to-toe examination for any other skin changes. I would examine for crepitus, any underlying fluctuance indicating drainable collections, mark the edges of the rash, and upload a photo to the patient record to help us monitor progression. I could use the finger-sweep test as an adjunct to my examination given my concerns about necrotising fasciitis. I would go back and re-assess the patient with an A–E approach to ensure they remain stable and to assess the effectiveness of any interventions I have started.

AAPS

Once happy with my assessment I would ensure the patient had suitable analgesia – necrotising fasciitis can be extremely painful. The ITU team should be ensuring a sufficient level of sedation and analgesia. I would urgently escalate concerns about potential necrotising fasciitis to my registrar on call, as well as ensuring we had senior ITU input in this case.

History, Notes, Investigations

I would ideally take an AMPLE history including the history of the rash and predisposing risk factors for necrotising fasciitis such as poorly controlled diabetes, other causes of immunosuppression, history of IVDU or skin trauma such as surgical interventions or insect bites. As the patient is intubated, this information will need to come from the primary team looking after the patient and the patient's notes, which should also be checked to determine trends in observations and bloods results.

Preliminary Management

The patient should be made nil by mouth and prepped for theatre (see 'Preparation for Theatre' below). A consent form 4 will need to be completed. Early discussion with microbiology about suitable antibiotic cover would also be prudent, as would discussing the situation with the patient's next of kin, given the high mortality of the condition.

Further Management

Intraoperatively, aggressive debridement of any necrotic and devitalised tissue down to healthy bleeding tissue with sending of samples (tissue and fluid) urgently for microbiology and histopathology should be performed. The wounds are often packed or temporised with a VAC (negative pressure vacuum) dressing and booked for relook in 24–48 hours depending on the patient's clinical status. Plastic surgery input will often be required for soft tissue coverage following resolution of infection. The patient will need careful post-operative monitoring on ITU.

Preparation for Theatre

It is essential you have a succinct paragraph explaining how you work up patients for CEPOD – you will need this in most scenarios. In this case the operation is class 1a (immediate life-saving).

> **CEPOD workup**
>
> *After discussing with my senior, I would prepare the patient for theatre by ensuring they were nil by mouth, consented by someone competent to do so, and marked. I would ensure they had all necessary preoperative investigations such as bloods (including clotting screen and group and saves), swabs (including COVID and MRSA), and an ECG. I would ensure they were booked onto the CEPOD list, and that I had alerted the theatre coordinator, anaesthetist on call, and the ward's nursing staff. I would discuss with ITU if there are concerns the patient may require critical care input postoperatively.*

How does necrotising fasciitis present? What intraoperative findings may be expected?
Necrotising fasciitis typically presents with rapidly progressing skin changes, a necrotic appearing purple/black rash, and with blisters or haemorrhagic bullae on oedematous skin. Crepitus may also be present. Patients are typically more systemically unwell than would be expected with a simple cellulitis. The patient may have risk factors (immunocompromised and diabetic patients, very frail or critically unwell patients) or precipitants (preceding

trauma/surgery, bites). Intraoperative findings include pus, easy separation of fascial planes, necrotic tissue, 'dishwater fluid' appearance, and vessel thrombosis.

What further investigations would you order to help diagnose necrotising fasciitis?
Necrotising fasciitis is a clinical diagnosis and while imaging such as USS, CT, or MRI may show air in the subcutaneous space, this should not delay urgent exploration and debridement in theatre. The 'finger sweep test' is a bedside diagnostic adjunct whereby a small incision is made over the affected area and a finger inserted. In necrotising fasciitis, the tissue dissects with minimal resistance, and 'dishwater fluid' is visible within the wound.

What is Fournier's gangrene?
Fournier's gangrene is a form of necrotising fasciitis affecting the perineal region. It has similar risk factors, presentation, and management as necrotising fasciitis elsewhere, but debridement should be performed by urology. General surgeons may be required if faecal diversion is required (e.g. formation of a stoma), and plastics may input regarding reconstruction.

9.3 Thoracic Trauma

You are the general surgical CT1 on call and are called to assess a 50-year-old male who has been brought to the emergency department following a high-speed road traffic accident. He has bruising across his chest and is gasping for air. Observations: RR 32, Sats 80% on RA, BP 90/60, HR 110, apyrexial. The trachea is deviated away from the side of the injury. How would you approach this patient?

Before you begin: This patient is extremely unwell; make sure a trauma call has been placed, your senior is aware, and necessary equipment is available. This is a thoracic trauma case, so having the ATOM-FC differential of life-threating chest pathology in your mind is essential (Airway obstruction or disruption, Tension pnuemothorax, Open pneumothorax, Massive haemothorax, Flail chest, Cardiac tamponade).

This patient is acutely unwell following a high-energy trauma. They should be managed in resus, a trauma call must be put out, and I would ensure my senior is aware of the case on my way down to review them. I would approach them using an ATLS A–E approach.

A–E

C-Spine
Given the high-energy trauma I would ensure the C-spine is triple immobilized until it can be cleared.

Airway
I would check for a patent, unobstructed airway using a look, listen, feel approach. I would look for cyanosis, accessory muscle use, tracheal tug, see-saw breathing, and visible signs of obstruction or penetrating airway trauma. I would listen for abnormal sounds such as grunting, snoring, gurgling, stridor and hoarseness of voice. I would feel for airflow out of the nose or mouth, and palpate the neck for any other evidence of obstruction. If I had any

concerns, I would ensure basic airway manoeuvres were conducted, the airway cleared of visible debris, and urgent anaesthetic review was performed.

Breathing

I would start 15 L of oxygen via a non-rebreather mask and ask a nurse to obtain a new set of observations including respiratory rate and oxygen saturations. I would assess for signs of respiratory distress or inadequate ventilation using an inspect, palpate, percuss, and auscultate approach. I would inspect for central cyanosis, neck vein distension, tracheal position, symmetry and quality of chest expansion, and paradoxical chest wall movement. I would palpate for rib tenderness and bilateral symmetrical chest expansion. I would auscultate for air entry bilaterally and added breath sounds such as wheezing or crepitations. This would help me evaluate potential causes of life-threatening chest pathology such as tension or open pneumothorax and massive haemothorax, which can present with similar clinical pictures.

Ongoing management of the pathology will depend on my clinical findings. Adjuncts such as ABG, CXR, and extended FAST scan are useful in these situations, but should not delay immediate lifesaving interventions such as needle decompression and chest drain for tension pneumothorax.

How this case proceeds from here depends on what life-threatening chest pathology is present. You may receive further information at some point to guide the assessment and management during your workup. If not, you should proceed to complete your full A–E assessment – more information may be provided once you are done.

The trachea is deviated away from the side of the injury and the side of the injury is hyper-resonant to percussion. How do you proceed?
This most likely represents a tension pneumothorax. This is a clinical diagnosis, which requires immediate needle decompression. The current ATLS approach advocates for decompression in the fourth or fifth intercostal space anterior to the mid-axillary line as this is more likely to reach the pleural space than inserting it into the midclavicular line second intercostal space [1]. Following this, I would reassess the patient from 'A' again. Chest drain insertion is required for definitive management. A portable CXR can be obtained urgently while the chest drain kit is being prepared, but this should not delay definitive management.

The trachea is central, breath sounds are reduced, and the lung is 'stony dull' to percussion, how do you proceed?
This likely represents haemothorax, which can be confirmed with chest X-ray or extended FAST scanning. The patient requires simultaneous volume resuscitation with warmed IV fluids followed by blood products as soon as they are available, and decompression of the chest cavity with a large bore chest tube (28–32 French). The volume of blood drained should be carefully monitored.

The drain is inserted and a large volume of blood drains. The patient remains haemodynamically unstable despite the drain and ongoing resuscitation, how do you proceed?
If the patient remains haemodynamically unstable despite resuscitation and decompression it is likely they will need to proceed urgently to emergency thoracotomy for surgical exploration and haemorrhage control. I would ensure there was ongoing resuscitation,

senior input, and begin to work the patient up for theatre (see Section 9.2 for theatre workup).

What defines a massive haemothorax?
A massive haemothorax is defined as a haemorrhage of more than 1500 ml blood (or one third the patient's total circulating volume) within the thorax. Accumulating this quantity on initial insertion of a chest drain, or ongoing drainage of more than 200 ml/hour for two to four hours, typically necessitates urgent thoracotomy.

The trachea is central, the patient is hypotensive, heart sounds are reduced, and the neck veins are distended; how do you proceed?
The triad of signs described is known as 'Beck's triad', which makes me concerned about the possibility of cardiac tamponade. Extended FAST scanning is a useful adjunct to confirm this as it is highly sensitive for detecting pericardial fluid in the hands of an experienced operator. ECG may show low voltage complexes. I would continue to resuscitate the patient, noting that IV fluids will raise the patient's venous pressure, which can improve cardiac output transiently while we await definitive management. This will come in the form of emergency thoracotomy or sternotomy. Ultrasound guided pericardiocentesis can be a further temporising measure while awaiting definitive management.

N.B. Kussmaul's sign (when breathing in the jugular venous pressure rises instead of falls) can also be a sign of tamponade, as can pulsus paradoxus (a drop in BP during deep inspiration). It is important to note that tamponade and tension pneumothorax can both present with shock and distension of neck veins, so examining the trachea and heart sounds is important, as is considering the mechanism of injury, and if able to, performing extended FAST scanning.

What are the boundaries of the triangle of safety for chest drain insertion?
Anterior: Lateral border of pectoralis major. Posterior: Anterior border of latissimus dorsi. Inferior: Fifth intercostal space.

Please describe the surgical technique for inserting a chest drain for a traumatic pneumothorax.
I would ensure I had all my equipment prepared, the patient was consented, there were no contraindications, and I had senior support on standby if required. I would position the patient on their back at 45 degrees with their hand behind their head. I would identify the triangle of safety. I would don sterile gloves and clean the area of insertion, apply drapes, and then inject local anaesthetic, infiltrating just above the inferior rib of the fifth intercostal space. I would anaesthetise the dermis and epidermis, then the intercostal muscles, periosteum, and pleura. I would make an incision parallel to the rib where the drain is to be inserted. Using large forceps I would use blunt dissection to pass through the subcutaneous tissues until the parietal pleura is breached. I would carefully insert a finger into the pleural cavity, perform a finger sweep, and make sure the lung is not adhered to the chest wall. I would insert the drain through the hole into the pleural cavity, aiming upwards, ensuring all holes along the drain are in the pleural space to avoid surgical emphysema. I would suture the drain in place, cover with a dressing, and attach the drain to an underwater drainage system and look for bubbling and swinging. I would request a post-procedure chest XR, provide further analgesia as required, and document the procedure.

How would you manage an open pneumothorax?

An open pneumothorax is a large open 'sucking chest wound'. If its diameter is more than two-third that of the trachea, then air preferentially goes via the wound during inspiration and into the pleural space:

I would place a sterile occlusive dressing over the wound which is impermeable to air and then seal it on only three sides to create a valve effect that lets air out during expiration but prevents it entering during inspiration. A chest drain is needed, as is definitive surgical closure of the wound.

Reference

1.   American College of Surgeons (2018). Committee on Trauma. ATLS: Student

Course Manual. Chicago, Ill.: American College of Surgeons.

9.4 Postoperative Shortness of Breath

A 72-year-old woman is day 2 following a hemiarthroplasty for a fractured neck of femur. The nurse calls you because the patient has become progressively more breathless throughout the morning. Her saturations have dropped to 87% and she has been placed on 4 L of nasal oxygen. She is tachycardic (107 bpm), BP: 161/90, RR: 20, temperature: 37.8°C. How would you approach this patient?

Before you begin: This case is about a fluent A–E, with a clear focus on the differential for postoperative shortness of breath (see below), so give 'breathing' enough focus in your A–E. As you are 'called by the nurse' you should provide instructions down the phone to help you for when you arrive at the bedside.

This patient sounds acutely unwell, and given her preceding immobility, I am particularly concerned about a possible pulmonary embolus, as well as the possibility of hospital-acquired pneumonia or COVID. I would go and assess them immediately using an A–E approach. Over the phone, I would ask the nursing staff to take a set of observations and prepare the patient's notes.

A–E

Airway

I would start by checking for a patent, unobstructed airway, initially by greeting the patient and assessing their ability to reply.

Breathing

I would then get an up-to-date respiratory rate and oxygen sats and start 15 L oxygen through a non-rebreather mask. I would then inspect, palpate, percuss, and auscultate the chest for signs of respiratory pathology. I would inspect for central cyanosis, neck vein distension, tracheal position, and symmetry and quality of chest expansion. I would auscultate for added breath sounds such as wheezing or crepitations, and for clearance of secretions when coughing. Given the patient is desaturating and feeling breathless, I would perform an ABG and consider a CXR.

Circulation

Once satisfied with her breathing, I would move on to assess circulation. I would ask the nurses to get an updated blood pressure and heart rate, examine the capillary refill time and radial pulses, and look for signs of peripheral overload. I would obtain IV access with a large bore cannula in each ACF. At this point I would take a full set of bloods including FBC, U&Es, clotting, and group and saves with a mind to any potential operative management, a VBG to get a rapid assessment of their Hb and lactate, and blood cultures if they are spiking a fever. In a hypotensive patient I would start a fluid bolus at this point as per CCRSIP guidelines. I would consider catheterising the patient and would get an ECG given they are tachycardic.

Disability

Once satisfied with my assessment and management of their circulation, I would examine the patient's neurological system with an AVPU score and pupillary examination, get a CBG, and check their temperature.

Exposure

I would then expose the patient, whilst preserving their dignity, to fully assess their respiratory and cardiovascular system. I would carefully consider their fluid status. I would examine the calves to check for signs of deep vein thrombosis.

AAPS

At this point, I reassess the patient to determine the effect of my interventions so far, and would offer analgesia and antiemetics, and alert my senior to my findings.

History, Notes, Investigation

I would take a focused history using an AMPLE structure before eliciting more information about the acuity of their respiratory symptoms, changes in sputum production, prior pulmonary pathology, and risk factors for VTE. I would examine the patient's operation notes, ward round entries since the operation, recent investigations, and the trend in their observations. I would also check their treatment escalation plan. I would check the drug chart to ensure appropriate VTE prophylaxis had been given. I would calculate a Wells' score for pulmonary embolism. I would then order further investigations as appropriate, including a COVID swab. A D-dimer may be considered based on their Well's score, but these are difficult to interpret in the perioperative period.

What is your differential diagnosis for postoperative SOB?

My differential can be split into infective causes (CAP, HAP, aspiration pneumonia, COVID, sepsis), ventilatory pathology (atelectasis, pulmonary oedema), and cardiovascular causes (PE, MI, fat embolism). There are also drug-related causes (ongoing action of NMJ blocking drugs, anaphylactic reactions) as well as shortness of breath secondary to pain or anxiety.

Given the limited information in the vignette, the most likely diagnoses on day 2 postoperatively would be pulmonary embolus, pneumonia, or basal atelectasis.

What is ERAS?

Enhanced Recovery After Surgery is a program introduced in the late 1990s to improve postoperative surgical outcomes using pre-, intra-, and postoperative interventions via the MDT. Preoperative interventions include preadmission counselling and patient education, nutritional support, and medical optimisation. Intraoperative interventions include minimally invasive surgery and minimising the use of drains. Postoperative interventions include early removal of tubes and catheters, early mobilisation, and pain control, minimising opioid use where possible.

What risk factors for postoperative respiratory complications do you know?

Non-modifiable risk factors include age, previous VTE, history of COPD, asthma, and OSA. Modifiable risk factors include smoking history, frailty and malnourishment (as identified by Rockwell and MUST scoring systems, respectively).

What scoring system might you use to assess the risk of a pulmonary embolus, and what investigations might you order?

I would use the Well's Criteria for PE. If the score was greater than 4, I would order an urgent CTPA and if this wasn't available within four to six hours, I would consider anticoagulating at therapeutic doses in the interim, after discussing with my seniors or haematology. If the score was 4 or less, I would conduct a D-dimer and if the result were raised, I would consider proceeding to CTPA. Otherwise, I would consider alternative diagnoses. However, I would be wary that in the perioperative period a D-dimer would be expected to be elevated, making this result harder to interpret.

The CTPA shows a sub-massive PE. The patient is haemodynamically stable. How would you manage this patient?

The definitive management in a haemodynamically stable patient is a minimum of three months of anticoagulation based on trust guidance, contraindications, comorbidities and patient preference. Therefore, I would reassess the patient with an A–E approach, ensure I had reviewed all investigations including clotting profile and renal profile, discuss the preferred anticoagulation options with the operating surgeon or one of my seniors, the pharmacist, and with the patient. The patient should be counselled appropriately, and I would ensure haematology follow-up is booked for review in three months.

Note that if the patient was shocked, invasive management with thrombolysis may be warranted – although her recent surgery would serve as a relative contraindication. Your role here would be to ensure the patient is appropriately resuscitated and then escalate to the operating surgeon, the medical team, the critical care outreach team, and haematology.

When would you opt for a V/Q scan instead of a CTPA?

V/Q scanning has similar sensitivity to CTPA, although CTPA is better able to detect clots in smaller vessels and is more likely to be available out of hours. CTPA will also give you more information regarding other likely differentials such as infection, atelectasis, and pulmonary oedema. V/Q scanning has the advantages of not needing contrast, and of providing a smaller radiation dose – of particular concern when scanning pregnant women as here the breast tissue absorbs a great deal of radiation from the CTPA.

9.5 Abdominal Trauma

You are the General surgical SHO on call and are called to assess a 19-year-old male patient who is being brought to resus by ambulance following a high-speed road traffic accident. He has abdominal bruising across the left upper quadrant and flank. He has a painful warm foot with abnormal angulation at the distal fibula. Observations are HR 125, BP 80/40, RR 26, Sats 98% on RA, apyrexial. How would you proceed?

Before you begin: Remember *life before limb* – do not be distracted by the limb, work through A–E methodically as this is the order in which things can be life threatening to the patient. Given the vignette, it is likely that 'circulation' is going to form the central focus of the scenario.

This haemodynamically unstable patient has suffered a high-energy trauma and from the information available appears extremely unwell. I would ensure a trauma call had been put out, and my senior was aware of the patient. I would proceed to assess the patient using an ATLS A–E approach.

A–E

C-Spine

Given the mechanism of injury, I would triple immobilise the C-spine with collar, blocks, and tape.

Airway

I would use a look, listen, feel approach to ensuring they have a patent unobstructed airway. If there are concerns about the ability of the patient to protect their airway, for example due to a reduced GCS, then we must ensure a definitive airway is established.

Breathing

I would assess for life-threatening respiratory pathology using an inspect, palpate, percuss, and auscultate approach. I would get up-to-date respiratory rate and oxygen sats. I would give the patient 15 L through a non-rebreather mask. I'd request adjuncts including ABG and portable chest X-ray as required.

Circulation

Once satisfied with breathing, I would assess the patient's haemodynamic status by checking central and peripheral capillary refill time, radial pulses, assessing the JVP and auscultating the precordium. I would get an up-to-date heart rate and blood pressure. I would ask an assistant to obtain wide bore IV access in both antecubital fossae. From one cannula I would ensure a full set of bloods (FBC, U&E, LFTs), a VBG (to check lactate and get a provisional Hb), clotting, group and saves (to cross match four units initially), and an amylase were taken. Into the other cannula I would ensure 1 L of warmed IV crystalloid fluid was given using a rapid infuser. Shock in the trauma setting is haemorrhage until proven otherwise and I would assess for signs of this in the chest, abdomen, pelvis, long bones, and for external haemorrhage. If the response to fluids was poor or there was concern regarding substantial bleeding, I would put out a major haemorrhage call and commence O negative blood transfusion. I would give one gram of tranexamic acid IV, place a pelvic binder if there were concerns about pelvic injury, and pack or apply pressure to any accessible source of bleeding.

Given the location of the bruising, I would be particularly worried about splenic injury. I would request a FAST scan to identify intra-abdominal bleeding quickly – the patient is currently too unstable to proceed to a CT scan. To complete my circulation workup, I would catheterise the patient to monitor urine output and consider an NG tube to decompress the stomach.

If the patient remains unstable despite fluid resuscitation and blood products, then the patient may require progression to emergency laparotomy: as blunt abdominal trauma with hypotension and a positive FAST scan would be an indication for laparotomy. The patient will need to be made NBM, and worked up for theatre with ongoing resuscitation, review by the general surgery registrar on call, anaesthetics on call, liaising with the theatre coordinator, ensuring any preoperative investigations are performed, booking into CEPOD and possibly booked for an ITU bed postoperatively.

N.B. at this point, the examiners may stop you at 'C' and ask you more questions (see below). More commonly you will get the opportunity instead to continue and complete your full assessment. If so, approach this as for previous scenarios, including working up the lower limb injury with a look, feel, move approach, radiological characterisation of the injury, and orthopaedic input. Examination of the limb is covered in Section 9.8.

If you cannot obtain IV access in the antecubital fossa, what would you do next?
I would ask a colleague to attempt to obtain peripheral IV access wherever they are able to do so, using ultrasound if required. If there were difficulties then alternatives such as intra-osseous access and ultrasound-guided large calibre central venous access (e.g. femoral, jugular, subclavian) should be obtained. This is patient and clinician skill dependent. This is why it is crucial for the trauma team leader to be aware of the competencies and experience of the team members.

Who/what does a major haemorrhage call activate?
The exact team this activates, and the composition of different blood packs, may vary by local centre, but the call will at the least typically alert anaesthetics/ICU, a porter, the blood bank, and the haematology team. A team member is nominated to be the contact for the blood bank. Initially you can give O negative blood until a group and save is completed. The first pack that is brought by the porter will often contain RBCs and

Table 9.1 Classes of shock

	Class I	Class II	Class III	Class IV
Blood loss	<750 ml (<15%)	750–1,500 ml (15%–30%)	1,500–2,000 ml (30%–40%)	>2,000 ml (>40%)
HR	<100	>100	>120	>140
BP	Normal	Normal	Decreased	Decreased
RR	14-20	20-30	30-40	>35
Mental status	Slightly anxious	Mildly anxious	Anxious and confused	Confused and lethargic

FFP, which are normally given in a fixed-ratio protocol to begin with. The second pack contains more RBCs, FFP, and PLTs. The transfusion protocol should be guided initially by local protocol, followed by coagulation results and liaison with haematology. In cases of massive transfusion a balanced ratio of RBC:FFP:PLT is often given.

What class of haemorrhagic shock is this patient in?
Based on the information in the scenario above they are likely in class III haemorrhagic shock. Table 9.1 is an adapted version from the Royal College of Emergency Medicine online learning module on shock [1].

What are the patterns of response to fluid therapy?
- Rapid response – patient becomes haemodynamically stable and maintenance fluids are required. Usually class I haemorrhage.
- Transient response – patient initially responds then deteriorate as fluids are slowed to maintenance levels (usually class II or III). Transfusion and definitive operative/interventional control of bleeding are needed.
- Minimal/no response – immediate definitive intervention is usually required to control major haemorrhage. Given this is unusual, do not forget to consider the other causes of shock.

What is the grading system for splenic injury? How are these injuries managed?
The American Association for the Surgery of Trauma (AAST) have produced injury scoring scales for different organ systems [2]. Splenic injuries are graded 1–5 based on the percentage of subcapsular haematoma surface area, depth of laceration, and associated vascular injury.

Management should be led by general surgeons and interventional radiologists, but typically angioembolisation is attempted in the first instance, but if this fails, or the patient is too haemodynamically unstable, then laparotomy ± splenectomy, or splenic salvage is required. Postoperatively the patient should be monitored for, and counselled regarding, thrombocytosis and overwhelming post-splenectomy infection with encapsulated bacteria (pneumococcus, meningococcus, and haemophilus influenzae type b). Lifelong vaccinations against these should be given, and prophylactic Pencillin V should be considered.

How would this case differ if the patient had RUQ bruising? What is the classification and management of liver injuries?
Workup would proceed in a similar management to the case above, with an emphasis on managing circulation before proceeding to a full top-to-toe examination. Similar to splenic injuries, AAST grades traumatic liver injuries 1–5. Grade is based on the percentage of subscapular haematoma, depth and length of parenchymal laceration, and the presence of associated parenchymal disruption and vascular injury.

Stable patients are usually managed conservatively with observation and serial examination, but in higher grade bleeds, angioembolisation may be attempted. If this fails, or the patient is unstable, then laparotomy is performed. Liver haemorrhage is controlled with manual compression, portal clamping, and perihepatic packing – sometimes left in place pending a re-look procedure – as well as direct liver suturing and coagulation.

References

1. RCEM (n.d.). 'Shock'. RCEM Learning, Website, www.rcemlearning.co.uk/reference/shock/#1571062626402-e8da7e9d-36a1.

2. American Association for the Surgery of Trauma. (n.d.). 'Injury Scoring Scales'. Website, www.aast.org/resources-detail/injury-scoring-scale#liver.

9.6 Testicular Pain

You are called to assess a 17-year-old man, brought in by ambulance due to sudden onset constant atraumatic pain in his right testicle for the last hour. His observations are stable. How would you approach this patient?

Before you begin: This is less likely to require a fully described A–E explanation. State that the most important differential is torsion early in your answer.

A–E

The history is concerning for possible testicular torsion. I would review the patient immediately and perform a thorough A–E assessment to ensure this patient was clinically stable and had no concurrent life-threatening pathology. Assuming there was no immediate concern from an A–E perspective, I would offer suitable analgesia and antiemetics, take a full focused clinical history, and examine the patient.

History and Examination

I would take an AMPLE history and a focused testicular history including trigger, onset, and duration of pain and any previous episodes of similar pain which might suggest intermittent torsion. I would ask about associated urinary symptoms and history of testicular trauma. I would take a full sexual history and history of previous scrotal operations, including previous orchidopexy. I would also elicit risk factors for testicular torsion, including family history, anatomical variants, such as Bell-Clapper testicles, and a history of undescended testicles. I would complete my history by taking a complete past medical, family, drug, allergy, and social history from the patient.

I would perform a full abdominal examination, including genito-scrotal and inguinal examination. Whilst the patient was standing, I would examine inguinal orifices to assess for hernias. Thereafter, I would inspect and palpate the testes with the patient lying on the bed. I would be looking for signs of torsion including a high riding, hard, swollen testicle with an abnormal lie, loss of the cremasteric reflex, and a negative Prehn's sign (elevating the testes does not improve the pain, unlike in epididymitis).

I could use a 'Testicular Workup for Ischaemia and Suspected Torsion' (TWIST) score to aid my clinical decision making in suspected torsion based on my history and examination findings.

I would send a urine dip ± MCS, a full set of bloods including FBC, U&Ss, CRP, and clotting, and obtain IV access.

Preliminary and Further Management

I would ensure the patient remained clinically stable. If I suspected torsion, I would urgently alert the urology registrar on call who will need to review the patient. The diagnosis in this case would ultimately be confirmed during scrotal exploration. I would ensure the patient was prepped for theatre – this case should ideally proceed to theatre within four to six hours of symptoms onset. I would inform my senior, the on-call anaesthetist, and the theatre coordinator about this case. I would ensure the patient has IV access, bloods, and fluids. I would make the patient nil-by-mouth, mark, and consent the patient for scrotal exploration ± bilateral orchidopexy ± orchidectomy ± proceed. I would provide the patient with a BAUS (British Association of Urological Surgeons) information leaflet.

Intraoperatively, my senior would perform scrotal exploration with orchidopexy of both testes if they are viable. If the viability is unclear, the testicle would be detorted and wrapped in a warm saline swab for 15 minutes before re-evaluating. During this time the contralateral testicle can be fixed if this is healthy. If viability remains unclear we could make a small stab incision through the tunica albuginea and look for bleeding. If the testicle is unsalvageable then an orchidectomy should be performed, with an orchidopexy to fix the contralateral side.

Would you request a testicular Doppler ultrasound for this patient?

I would not request a Doppler ultrasound unless it would not delay the patient going to theatre. A negative Doppler does not preclude the need for operative exploration.
An ultrasound is more useful to confirm other diagnoses in acute scrotal pain such as epididymo-orchitis or scrotal abscess.

What is the pathophysiology of testicular torsion?

Twisting of the spermatic cord results in impaired venous return and oedema, which eventually impedes arterial inflow, causing ischaemia and then infarction of the testicle.

What is your differential diagnosis for acute scrotal pain?

A useful acronym in these situations is HIINNT:

> Hernia: strangulated inguinoscrotal hernia
> Ischaemia: testicular torsion, torsion of the testicular appendage, testicular infarction
> Infectious: acute epididymo-orchitis, viral orchitis, scrotal abscess, infected hydrocoele
> Neoplastic: tumour with infection/bleed/infarct
> Non-scrotal: renal colic with radiating pain
> Trauma: ruptured testicle, intratesticular haematoma

What are the complications of a missed testicular torsion?

Testicular infarction risk increases rapidly with each passing hour; after 24 hours the rate of salvage is less than 10%. A patient with torsion should aim to be taken to theatre within six hours of pain onset and this is an NCEPOD class 1b case. Late complications of a missed torsion include abscess or sinus formation, formation of anti-sperm antibodies causing infertility in the contralateral testis, and risk of torsion in the contralateral testis.

What are the complications of scrotal exploration and orchidopexy?
As for all procedures, there are risks of infection, bleeding, acute pain, damage to surrounding structures and anaesthetic risks. Specific risks for this procedure include a need for orchidectomy, chronic scrotal pain, discomfort from patients feeling stitches through the skin, late atrophy of the testicle, and reduced fertility.

9.7 Acute Abdominal Pain

You are the on-call general surgical SHO at a DGH overnight. You are called to the emergency department to assess a 75-year-old male smoker who has presented with severe sudden onset abdominal pain. He looks pale. Observations are HR 160, BP 90/65, RR 16, Sats 98% on RA. They are afebrile. How do you proceed?

Before you begin: Abdominal pain and shock in an elderly man is a ruptured abdominal aortic aneurysm (AAA) until proven otherwise. However, the differential is very broad (see below), so reference this, while still stressing the urgency of the situation: it is often said that of patients with a ruptured AAA, 50% won't make it to hospital, and of those that do, 50% will unfortunately never leave.

As discussed in the Introduction, as answers become bullet points, basic information (such as how to assess an airway in this scenario) are excluded from the model answer. It is expected that you will have developed and memorised your own script for these and they be included in your answer, and the A–E we provide is more focused on the specific details pertinent to the case at hand.

A–E
Airway
Breathing
Circulation

- Large bore IV access in both antecubital fossae, full set of bloods including FBC, U&Es, clotting, group and saves (and cross match six units or more initially), and a VBG for a rapid assessment of hgb and lactate. Activate the major haemorrhage protocol if there are concerns about AAA rupture and get anaesthetic, critical care, and vascular support immediately.
- Fluid resuscitation in cases of ruptured AAA should be aiming for 'permissive hypotension', as posterior rupture of an AAA can lead to transient tamponade of bleeding due to formation of a haematoma within a closed space. Aim for a mean arterial pressure between 60 and 80 mmHg to maintain cerebral perfusion without worsening the bleeding.
- Examine for source of bleeding, including assessing the abdomen for signs of AAA or retroperitoneal bleeding.
- ECG as the patient is tachycardic.
- Catheterise.

Disability
Exposure

- Examine for signs of vascular disease: lower limb pulses, signs of peripheral aneurysm, signs of lower limb ischaemia ('Trash foot').

AAPS

- Urgent senior involvement; note that you should be getting senior involvement immediately upon assessing the patient. Vascular surgery, anaesthetics, and the critical care outreach team should be involved from the start.

History, Notes, Investigation

- AMPLE structure looking also for vasculopathy risk factors.
- If the patient is unstable, or CT cannot be immediately performed, a FAST scan can help confirm the diagnosis – the patient must proceed to theatre if they are not stabilised.
- If the patient is stable, NICE recommends a CT aortogram as the gold standard. This will also allow preoperative EVAR (stent-graft) planning.

Preliminary Management

- Resuscitation as above and begin workup for emergency theatre (see Section 9.2). A ruptured AAA is CEPOD classification 1a – immediate life threatening.

Further Management

- Ruptured AAAs require definitive surgical management. Repairs can be performed using an open approach or an endovascular approach depending on the patient's fitness, anatomy of the AAA, and the institutional expertise.
- Postoperatively, the patient will usually require intensive care admission.
- Postoperative care includes smoking cessation, obtaining a healthy weight, and vascular-protective medications including a statin, aspirin, and anti-hypertensives.
- If EVAR is performed they will need ongoing lifelong surveillance of their stent-graft.

What are the differentials for abdominal pain in this patient?
It is important to use a systems-based differential – this shows you can categorise your thoughts appropriately and will make it much easier to think of a list in the heat of the moment. The box below demonstrates a comprehensive systems-based approach to abdominal pain. Pick around a half dozen of the most likely differentials – do not reel off this entire list!

Abdominal pain differential by system:

- Vascular causes: ruptured AAA, symptomatic AAA (impending rupture), acute aortic dissection
- Renal causes: ureteric colic, pyelonephritis
- Upper GI causes: perforated peptic ulcer, pancreatitis, gallbladder disease
- Lower GI causes: bowel perforation, bowel ischemia, perforated diverticulitis, appendicitis, IBD, hernia-related pathology
- MSK: fractures, muscular/ligamentous causes
- Gynae: ovarian torsion/rupture, ectopic pregnancy, Mittelschmerz
- Medical: DKA, cardiovascular pathology such as MI, respiratory pathology such as PE

What risk factors are there for AAA?

The most common risk factor is smoking. Risk factors can be split into non-modifiable (age, male sex, family history, history of connective tissue disorders or previous dissection) and modifiable (smoking, hypertension, high cholesterol). Diabetes, although a risk factor for atherosclerotic disease, is relatively protective for aneurysmal disease. Remember that patients can develop mycotic aneurysms (typically from salmonella, TB, or syphilis), vasculitic aneurysms, and traumatic aneurysms too.

What screening is available for AAAs in the UK?

Since 2013, all men have been offered screening with a one-off abdominal ultrasound at age 65. If their abdominal aortic diameter is >3 cm, they enter ongoing ultrasound surveillance (3–4.4 cm: yearly surveillance, 4.5–5.4 cm: three-monthly surveillance, >5.5 cm: two-week wait referral for vascular surgical consultation). Surgery is typically offered for aneurysms >5.5 cm, those which have grown >0.5 cm in six months, or patients who are symptomatic.

When would a patient be considered for an endovascular repair (EVAR) vs an open repair

While this is a decision for senior vascular surgeons and radiologists to make, a general principle is that endovascular procedures are typically more suitable for frail or comorbid patients. Endovascular procedures also require anatomy congruent for a stent-graft. These patients will require lifetime follow-up and have a higher rate of secondary interventions. Open procedures 'frontload' the operative risk to the first few weeks – but it is less common to need to re-intervene in these patients. This may be more appropriate in younger, fitter patients.

What complications would you warn patients about for AAA surgery?

All surgical procedures have a risk of bleeding, infection, damage to surrounding structures, thromboembolic risks, anaesthetic risks, scarring, failure, and need for a repeat/further procedure. Additionally, there are specific risks for this procedure. These may be immediate (such as spinal cord ischaemia), early (such as AKI, MI, stroke, gut ischaemia and trash foot), or late (anastomotic pseudoaneurysm, endovascular leak – if EVAR used).

9.8 Acutely Painful Leg

You are called to review a 65-year-old woman who has come to the emergency department complaining of a six-hour history of atraumatic severe right leg pain. She is a diabetic, has raised cholesterol, and smokes 20 cigarettes a day. How do you proceed?

Before you begin: Important differentials include acute limb ischaemia (ALI), a DVT, or compartment syndrome. Her comorbidities make ALI more likely. Other causes would include gout or cellulitis. A straightforward well-rehearsed A–E should allow plenty of time to get to the additional questions.

A–E

Airway
Breathing
Circulation

- Bloods including VBG, clotting screen, FBC, U&Es, and group and saves as part of a preoperative workup.

– ECG to assess for AF given possible embolic causes of acute limb ischaemia.

Disability
– Stress that you would monitor CBGs given the diabetes history.

Exposure
– Complete vascular examination of the lower limbs using a look/feel/move approach to identify the '6 P's' of limb ischaemia (pain, pallor, paraesthesia, perishingly cold, pulselessness, paralysis). Signs of tissue loss include gangrene, pallor, and mottling – fixed non-blanching mottling is a sign of irreversible limb ischaemia.
– Examine for signs of other vascular aneurysms, including AAA and popliteal aneurysm.

N.B. the examination of a limb is an important one to be able to describe completely and succinctly. Practising this is essential. For example:

> **Limb examination**
>
> *I would examine the limb using a look, feel, move approach, exposing both legs to compare the two sides. I would inspect for asymmetry, deformity, angulation, open wounds, erythema, pallor, discolouration, and swelling. I would palpate for tenderness, swelling, distal pulses, capillary refill time, neurological status, and temperature. A Doppler probe is a useful adjunct to assess the pulses. I would assess active and passive movement of the limb, being wary of the potential for this to be extremely painful. I would ensure neurovascular status was documented.*

AAPS
– Opioid analgesia will likely be required. This patient should be urgently escalated to your senior.

History, Notes, Investigations
– AMPLE history with identification of vascular risk factors and features pointing to thrombotic vs embolic causes.
– Handheld Doppler assessment at the bedside to examine pulses.
– Depending on access to scans, options include MR angiogram, CT angiography and arterial duplex (US). MR angiogram is first line if available, as per NICE guidance. CT angiography is faster and more readily available. These are particularly helpful for establishing whether a thrombus extends to the aortoiliac segment. An arterial duplex is cheaper, does not require contrast, but is highly operator dependent, often unavailable out of hours, and will struggle to evaluate the aorto-iliac segment.

Preliminary Management
– Resuscitation with fluids and high-flow oxygen, preoperative workup for CEPOD (see Section 9.2).

Your investigations reveal the patient has acute limb ischaemia; please outline the management options for this patient.
I would divide the further management options into medical, endovascular, and open surgical. A Rutherford score can help determine prognosis while determining the extent of

ischaemia, and the underlying cause (thrombotic vs embolic) helps guide management (Table 9.2). *Medical options include anticoagulation, typically with IV heparin boluses followed by heparin infusions based on activated partial thromboplastin time (APTT) measurements. Endovascular options include local intra-arterial thrombolysis, and angioplasty. Surgical options include arteriotomy and embolectomy, and surgical bypass procedures. Cases that undergo revascularisation should also be considered for four compartment fasciotomy due to the risk of compartment syndrome. Finally, irreversible limb ischaemia will require amputation or palliation. Long-term, the patient will require cardiovascular risk factor management with exercise, smoking cessation, weight loss, lipid lowering management, as well as long-term anti-thrombotics.*

What are the causes of acute limb ischaemia?
Roughly 80 per cent of ALI cases are caused by acute thrombosis in situ on the background of atherosclerotic vessel disease. Around 20 per cent are caused by embolic causes, typically from AF or other cardiac causes such as recent MI or heart valve pathology. There are also rarer causes such as trauma, a dissecting aneurysm, and stent-graft thrombosis.

What are the differences between thrombotic and embolic causes?

Table 9.2 Factors to differentiate embolic from thrombotic causes of ALI

	Embolic	Thrombotic
Onset	Seconds – minutes	Hours – days
History	Risk factors for embolic sources, e.g. AF	Previous claudication, vasculopath risk factors, signs of CLI on contralateral side, previous vascular surgery
Examination	Contralateral leg pulses present Bruits absent Soft artery on palpation	Contralateral leg pulses absent Bruits present Calcified artery on palpation

What classification systems are available to estimate limb viability?
The Rutherford classification can be used (Table 9.3). As a rough guide, Rutherford I + IIA may be amenable to trial of heparin (infusion) in the first instance while IIB typically proceeds to operative management.

How does unfractionated heparin work?
Unfractionated heparin is an activator of antithrombin leading to inactivation of factor Xa and thrombin and therefore is an antagonist of factor Xa. Heparin has an advantage over other anticoagulants in acute settings as it produces systemic anticoagulation almost immediately and can be rapidly reversed with protamine.

How is ankle-brachial pressure index (ABPI) measured? How are these scores interpreted?
ABPI is the ratio of systolic blood pressure in the ankle to that in the arm, providing information about blood flow in the lower limbs. To perform ABPI you should place

Table 9.3 Rutherford classification of ALI

Category	Description	Sensory loss	Muscle weakness	Arterial Doppler	Venous Doppler
I	Viable/no immediate threat	None	None	Audible	Audible
IIA	Marginally threatened – salvageable is treated quickly	Minimal (toes)	None	Inaudible	Audible
IIB	Immediately threatened – salvageable with immediate revascularisation	More than toes	Mild to moderate	Inaudible	Audible
III	Irreversible/permanent tissue or nerve damage inevitable	Profound	Profound	Inaudible	Inaudible

Source: Adapted from Rutherford et al. [1].

the blood pressure cuff on the upper arm, identify the brachial pulse with a hand-held Doppler, inflate the cuff to occlude the signal, then slowly deflate to determine the pressure at which the arterial signal is audible again. Repeat for the contralateral arm and document the higher of the readings. Repeat this with the cuff on the left and right ankles (assessing posterior tibial artery and dorsalis pedis arteries with a hand-held Doppler), taking the highest of the readings for each ankle. Divide each ankle's highest score by the highest of the brachial scores to calculate a left and right ABPI. A score of 0.9–1.4 is considered normal, 0.8–0.9 indicates mild disease, 0.5–0.8 indicates moderate disease, <0.5 indicates significant disease. Note that a score >1.4 usually represents vessel calcification in the context of diabetes.

What is the surface anatomy for points of arterial palpation on the lower limb?
- Dorsalis pedis: lateral to extensor hallucis longis tendon.
- Posterior tibial: halfway between posterior aspect of medial malleolus and insertion of the Achilles tendon.
- Popliteal: inferior aspect of popliteal fossa with slightly flexed knee.
- Femoral: mid-inguinal point (ASIS to pubic symphysis).

Reference

1. Rutherford RB, Baker JD, Ernst C, Johnston KW, Porter JM, Ahn S, Jones DN (1997). 'Recommended standards for reports dealing with lower extremity ischemia: Revised version'. *Journal of Vascular Surgery* 26(3): 517–538, https://doi.org/10.1016/s0741-5214(97)70045-4.

9.9 Abdominal Distension

You are the general surgical CT1 and have been called to review a 57-year-old woman who has presented with abdominal pain and multiple episodes of vomiting. There is no blood in her vomitus. Her past medical history is notable for previous open salpingo-oophorectomy. Her observations are HR 105, BP 105/90, RR 16, Sats 96% on room air, and she is afebrile.

Before you begin: Abdominal pain and vomiting with a history of major open abdominal surgery should make you concerned for bowel obstruction (namely adhesional small bowel obstruction). This is a common condition, and most candidates can describe a passable approach to this scenario. To stand out, top candidates should have a smooth approach and a more impressive depth of knowledge. Your assessment can demonstrate that you understand the differentials without being asked directly. You will often be able to work out the answer from the stem, but you should answer as though you have a broad differential in mind.

A–E
Airway
Breathing
- A distended abdomen can splint the diaphragm and impair inspiration, if there are concerns about inspiration then an ABG and CXR would be appropriate first steps.

Circulation
- The patient is tachycardic and hypotensive. The bowel produces around 9 L of fluid/day in an adult, and fluid losses in bowel obstruction can be significant. Begin fluid resuscitation and catheterise to monitor fluid balance.
- Full set of bloods (see below) with a mind to potential operative management and to identify electrolyte disturbances which may be causes of altered bowel movement. A VBG to assess for lactate and provide a rapid assessment of the patient's hgb.
- Given patient is tachycardic – ECG.

Surgical bloods
- FBC, U&Es, LFT, CRP are almost universally ordered and are easily justified. If questioned, a fall-back answer is to say they establish a baseline to help monitor the patient's progression. Amylase and bone profile can also be considered based on the case at hand.
- Clotting and group and saves are required in cases proceeding to theatre and all cases involving haemorrhage.
- A VBG is useful in almost all cases and provides a rapid assessment of a patient's hgb, as well as their lactate and electrolytes.
- Blood cultures in any infective pathology.

Disability
- Check glucose – patient likely to have had impaired oral intake in the preceding hours/days.

Exposure

- Full head-to-toe examination with a focused abdominal examination to check for scars, peritonism, distension, a tympanic abdomen, and tinkling bowel sounds.
- PR examination to check for faecal impaction, or an empty rectum in obstruction.
- Hernial orifices to ensure no incarcerated/strangulated hernias as cause of obstruction.

AAPS

- Patients will require analgesia but be wary of giving excessive analgesia that slows bowel motility, such as opiates. Avoid prokinetic antiemetics if there is a complete mechanical obstruction – the intestine can squeeze against this block and worsen the pain.

History, Notes, Investigation

- AMPLE history to determine the timescale of vomiting, failure to pass stool/flatus, and nausea, to help characterise large bowel obstruction (constipation precedes nausea and vomiting) vs small bowel obstruction (nausea and vomiting precede constipation). For cases of bowel obstruction, determining the aetiology is also helpful – take a full GI history including previous operations which may predispose to adhesional SBO, previous hernias, weight loss, recent change in bowel habit, and family history of cancer.
- Radiological investigations including erect CXR, AXR, and CT abdomen pelvis with contrast should be considered (see below).

Preliminary and Further Management

- Resuscitation with IV fluids, NBM with an NGT on free drainage with four hourly aspirates. N.B. 'drip and suck' refers to IV fluids coupled with Ryles tube insertion to decompress the stomach.
- Definitive management will vary based on the underlying aetiology. A 24–48 hour trial of conservative management is appropriate for adhesional SBO without signs of ischaemia, strangulation, or perforation. Gastrografin may be used during this time as a clinical adjunct (see below).
- In cases where this has failed, where there are signs of bowel ischaemia, closed loop obstruction, or an extrinsic cause such as a tumour, operative management will most likely be required. In which case the patient needs preparation for theatre.
- If there are concerns about nutritional state, dietician review should be requested.

The patient became nauseous and started vomiting 18 hours ago. She has not opened her bowels in six hours. What is the most likely cause of the underlying pathology?
The clinical picture provided points towards SBO, with her history of abdominal procedures making an adhesional SBO the most likely cause. This is the most common cause of SBO, followed by hernias.

How would you categorise the causes of bowel obstruction in general?
There are intraluminal causes such as an impacted foreign body, gallstone ileus, and faecal impaction, intramural causes such as malignancy, inflammatory stricture, radiation enteritis, and intussusception, and extraluminal causes such as adhesions, incarcerated hernias, and peritoneal metastases.

Would you get an abdominal and erect chest X-ray or proceed directly to CT abdomen pelvis?
While previously AXR and erect CXR formed an important initial assessment, CT is more sensitive, demonstrates the cause and level of the obstruction, and helps diagnose bowel ischaemia. The ASGBI small bowel obstruction pathway recommends CT over AXR for all but frequent attenders with a benign clinical picture, as plain radiography is less sensitive and less reliable [1].

What role does gastrografin have in adhesional SBO?
Gastrografin has both a diagnostic and therapeutic role. It is a high osmolar radio-opaque water-soluble contrast medium which causes fluid to be drawn into the bowel lumen, reducing bowel wall oedema and helping to stimulate peristalsis. It can be given in adhesional SBO, after which the NGT should be spigotted, and a repeat abdominal XR performed six hours later. If contrast reaches the ileocecal valve/large colon within six hours, it implies that the SBO is likely to resolve. Failure of contrast to reach the colon implies surgical intervention is more likely to be needed.

The patient is diagnosed with adhesional small bowel obstruction but does not progress with a trial of 24-hour conservative management. An operation is planned. What would you consent the patient for?
I would always clarify with the operating surgeon what operation they would like the patient consented for, and ensure I felt competent in consenting the patient for this. Likely operations in this instance would be laparoscopy ± adhesiolysis ± small bowel resection ± stoma formation ± conversion to open ± proceed. It is important the patient is fully consented for possible outcomes preoperatively: in this situation, covering for the possibility that an area of necrotic bowel needing resection and stoma formation is essential. A stoma nurse review, where stoma formation is a possibility, is always sensible.

How would your management change if the patient was an elderly multimorbid frail patient presenting with sigmoid volvulus?
Sigmoid volvulus is a form of large bowel obstruction caused by the bowel rotating on its mesentery. This typically presents in the constipated, multimorbid elderly patient. The initial workup would be similar, being wary of the effects of large fluid shifts in a frail patient. AXR classically shows a 'coffee bean' sign. After appropriate resuscitation, most patients are managed with a rectal tube placed with the aid of a rigid sigmoidoscope. This tube may remain in for 24 hours while the bowel decompresses. The patient is observed for two to three days to ensure there is no bowel ischaemia, which gives time to address possible precipitating factors (medication adjustments, mobility work, changing care set up at home). If a rectal tube does not work, or if the patient has signs of ischaemia or perforation, then operative management for resection of the redundant sigmoid loop with primary anastomosis or colostomy may be required.

How would your management change if the patient was an elderly patient presenting in pseudo-obstruction

Pseudo-obstruction is a differential in cases of large bowel obstruction. It refers to dilatation of the large bowel caused by altered peristalsis without mechanical obstruction. Workup would be similar to the above. Conservative management (drip and suck), correcting any electrolyte abnormalities and treating any underlying causes is appropriate in most cases. If this fails, neostigmine can be used in some cases to increase peristalsis. Invasive approaches include decompression with rectal tube, and surgery if there are signs of perforation or ischaemia. A comprehensive geriatric assessment would be appropriate to identify and manage possible underlying causes, including neurological conditions such as Parkinson's, polypharmacy with opioids, and electrolyte imbalances.

How would your management change if the patient was an otherwise fit and healthy 55-year-old man who is in large bowel obstruction secondary to an obstructing colonic tumour?

In this situation, conservative management is inappropriate; resection, stenting, or defunctioning with a stoma is required. Workup and resuscitation will be similar but operative management will depend on intraoperative findings. Typically, those below the peritoneal reflection should have the colon defunctioned via a stoma, followed by staging, MDT discussion, and definitive management at a later date. Attempting to resect low tumours like these in the emergency setting is rarely undertaken due to the risk of positive circumferential margins. Higher tumours (e.g. rectosigmoid) are sometimes managed with a Hartmann's procedure, where the tumour area is resected, the distal rectal stump is closed, and an end colostomy is brought out. In the interview, it is important to mention that this case would be managed with an MDT approach, keeping the patient's wishes at the heart of the management plan, and ensuring the patient's physical, social, and psychological needs are attended to. An understanding of the basic principles of surgical management in these cases is enough – these are senior decisions!

Reference

1. Association of Surgeons of GB (n.d.). 'SBO National Pathway'. Website, 19 Feb. 2024, www.asgbi.org.uk/emergency-general-surgery/sbo-national-pathway#:~:text=A%20National%20pathway%20to%20improve.

9.10 Testicular Lump

You are the Urology CT1 on call and are asked to come to the urgent care centre to assess a 17-year-old man with a growing painless lump on his left testicle. The patient is clinically well, speaking normally, and not in pain. Observations are stable. Routine blood tests are normal. How would you approach this patient?

Before you begin: This is a patient with a stable presentation and the A–E assessment should therefore be brief. The key to this presentation is working through a thorough scrotal exam and having a clear differential.

A–E

This patient appears well. I would assess the patient with a CCRISP-guided A–E approach to ensure the patient was stable. If there were any aberrations in my A–E assessment, I would treat these first, before proceeding to a focused history and examination of the inguino-scrotal region.

History and Examination

I would begin by taking a comprehensive history of the lump, including the site, when it developed, if it has changed in size, and any associated pain, tethering, recent trauma, or lower urinary tract symptoms. I would also ask about systemic features such as fever, anorexia/malaise/weight loss, gynaecosmastia, as well as signs of metastases, such as shortness of breath, lymphadenopathy, back pain, or neurological symptoms. It is also important to gather a complete sexual history and past medical and surgical history, looking in particular for previous testicular malignancy, history of undescended testis, infections, or infertility, and a family history of testicular cancer.

I would perform a general examination feeling for supraclavicular nodes, examining the chest and abdomen looking for any scars from childhood orchidopexy. I would then perform a scrotal examination including examining the testicles, epididymis, spermatic cord, and regional lymph nodes. I would then focus on the lump and characterise the site, size, shape, consistency, tenderness, temperature, transillumination, and tethering of the lump, comparing to the contralateral size. I would try to get above the lump, check the cough impulse, and see if the lump can be reduced. I would note the presence of any varicocoele.

Preliminary Management

This stable patient with a scrotal lump should be investigated with a urine dip, blood tests including inflammatory markers and tumour markers (beta-HCG, alpha-fetoprotein, LDH), and an urgent testicular ultrasound. In the acute setting, ordering these investigations and referring the patient for urgent follow-up in clinic would be sufficient. The patient should be safety-netted, including to return if they develop acute severe scrotal pain or infective symptoms.

Further Management

This would depend on the likely diagnosis (see below). Infectious causes should be managed with antibiotics or incision and drainage for an abscess. If malignancy is suspected a CT CAP scan would be organised to stage the disease, and the patient would be referred to the MDT. Biopsy is not generally performed, instead, histology is analysed after a radical inguinal orchidectomy. Semen banking may be considered prior to surgery. Subsequent management should be determined by the MDT but generally involves surveillance and/or chemotherapy.

What is your differential for a unilateral scrotal lump?
I would classify lumps as testicular, extra-testicular, and extra-scrotal. Testicular causes include tumours, torsion, and abscesses. Extra-testicular causes include hydrocoele, varicocoele, spermatocoele, haematocoele, epididymal cyst, epididymitis, previous surgical

intervention (e.g. sutures from orchidopexy), sebaceous cysts, TB, and syphilis (both rare). Extra-scrotal causes include inguinal hernia.

N.B. if the scenario is a painful testicular lump, recall that a minority of testicular tumours present with a dull ache, and a smaller minority can present with acute pain. Therefore, they should not be completely neglected in your differential.

What are the risk factors for testicular cancer?
Modifiable risk factors include infections such as HIV, HPV, and EBV, as well as testicular trauma. Non-modifiable risk factors include cryptorchidism, personal and familial history of testicular cancer, and infertility.

9.11 Head Injury in Trauma

You are the orthopaedic CT1 and are called to assess a 65-year-old woman who has just arrived in resus following a high-speed road traffic accident. She has bruising and superficial bleeding around her head. She is opening her eyes to pain, babbling inappropriate words, and withdrawing from pain. Her observations are currently stable. How would you approach this patient?

Before you begin: A drop in GCS in the context of a head injury is very concerning. Work the patient up using your trauma A–E. While reading the vignette, calculate a GCS score where the information to work this out is available – it will almost certainly be important or asked about later. Again, this is not a case you should be managing alone, and senior input should be sought from the start.

A–E
C-Spine
– Triple immobilise the C-spine with collar, blocks, and tape.

Airway
– Close assessment of the airway to assess patency. GCS of 8 or lower typically requires intubation by anaesthetics. Note that sedative or paralytic agents should be avoided where possible until GCS has been examined as these may interfere with GCS measurements. The GCS should be regularly re-evaluated as it can drop during the assessment, in which case the airway must be re-evaluated.

Breathing
Circulation
– The patient should be haemodynamically stabilised aiming for systolic BP $\geq$110 mmHg (>100 if aged 50–70).
– If the systolic blood pressure cannot be raised >100 mmHg then identifying the cause takes priority over neurological evaluation – intracranial injury alone is unlikely to cause haemorrhagic shock.

Disability
– Perform a focused neurological examination for GCS, pupillary responses, and focal neurology. From the clinical information above, her GCS is 9 (E2V3M4). TBI is classified into mild (GCS 13–15), moderate (GCS 9–12), and severe (GCS 3–8).

Remember to use the patient's best responses when calculating GCS. Serial neurological examinations must be performed.

- Temperature and CBG.
- Consider blood alcohol level and toxicology screen for those with TBI.
- Determine need for CT head as per NICE guidelines (clearly it will be needed here).

Exposure

- Full top-to-toe examination including log roll.

AAPS

- Shorter-acting analgesia is preferable to minimise interference with GCS calculations. Senior support would be essential in this case.

History, Notes, Investigations

- A patient with a reduced GCS is unlikely to provide a full AMPLE history but try to obtain this from another source.
- CT trauma (including head and neck) is required. The patient must have a safe airway before proceeding to scanning. While every effort should be made to scan the head, this technically should not delay transfer of the patient to a trauma centre that is capable of immediate and definitive neurosurgical intervention if this is required. It also does not take priority over taking a patient for emergency laparotomy/ thoracotomy for major haemorrhage management.

Preliminary Management

- Discussion with neurosurgery to determine ongoing management.
- In the interim, secondary brain injury can be minimised by maintaining a blood pressure sufficient for cerebration and keeping the patient normothermic, normoglycaemic, and correcting coagulopathy.
- In cases of severe TBI, temporising measures such as mannitol, hypertonic saline, or periods of brief hyperventilation can be used to temporarily reduce intracranial pressure prior to definitive management. These measures should only be done with neurosurgical and anaesthetic/ITU input.
- IV broad spectrum antibiotics for all open skull fractures.
- As per the latest NICE guidance, consider giving a 2 g bolus of tranexamic acid as soon as possible (within two hours) in patients >16 years old who have moderate or severe TBI [1].

Further Management

- This will depend on the underlying pathology. Very broadly, mild TBI (GCS 13–15) requires neurosurgery discussion if there are abnormalities on CT scan or the patient is deteriorating. Moderate TBI (GCS 9–12) usually needs neurosurgical review (depending on CT findings), ATLS workup, and follow-up CT in 12–24 hours. Severe TBI (GCS 3–8) typically requires urgent neurosurgical transfer following intubation and ventilation to manage underlying pathology. For example, craniotomy and haematoma evacuation in the case of a large epidural haematoma.

During the CT scan the patient deteriorates further. They are now not opening their eyes, babbling random sounds, and withdrawing from pain. How would you manage this patient now?

This patient has had their GCS drop to 7. Therefore, they need an urgent repeat anaesthetic review of their airway for consideration of intubation and ventilation; if they are currently still protecting their airway, they may not be for long. Work the patient up as before and seek urgent neurosurgical input.

What is a definitive airway?

A cuffed tube in the trachea, with the cuff sitting below the level of the vocal cords.

What are the criteria for CT head in head injury in adults?

NICE updated its guidance on the management of head trauma in 2023. The CT head criteria are worth learning [1]. CT head should be performed within one hour if: GCS <13 on initial assessment or <15 after two hours, signs of open/depressed/basal skull fractures, post-traumatic seizure, >1 vomit since the episode, or focal neurological deficit. CT should occur within 8 hours if the patient is >65 years old, has a bleeding or clotting disorder, is involved in a dangerous mechanism of injury, or has more than 30 minutes' retrograde amnesia of events immediately before the head injury. If a patient presents greater than eight hours after the incident, you should perform the CT within one hour. You should consider a CT head within eight hours of the incident in those on anticoagulation or antiplatelets.

In a patient with mild TBI, who is suitable for discharge, how would you safety-net the patient?

Safety-net the patient to return if: they lose consciousness, have a seizure, begin vomiting, develop signs of CSF leak, develop a reduced GCS or develop focal neurology such as weakness, loss of sensation, and pupil abnormalities. They should be warned about not drinking or taking sedatives. The risk and benefit of restarting any anti-thrombotics should be discussed. The patient should be discharged with a reliable companion at home.

What clinical signs indicate a base of skull fracture?

Haemotympanum, raccoon eyes, Battle's sign, CSF leak (rhinorrhoea or otorrhoea).

What is Cushing's triad?

A physiological response to raised intracranial pressure leads to Cushing's triad of a widened pulse pressure, bradycardia, and irregular respirations. This is due to an initial sympathetic and then parasympathetic overstimulation. Hypertension occurs to help maintain cerebral perfusion.

Reference

1. NICE (2023). 'Overview | Head injury: Assessment and early management | Guidance | NICE'. Website, www.nice.org.uk, www.nice.org.uk/guidance/ng232.

9.12 Post-thyroidectomy Swelling

You are the ENT CT1 on call overnight. While walking through the ward you notice a breathless patient who is four hours post total thyroidectomy. They are pointing at their neck where there is significant swelling. They are unable to speak and are clearly extremely distressed. How do you proceed?

Before you begin: Given the recent total thyroidectomy, you are concerned about an evolving haematoma in the anterior neck compressing the airway. Leave your examiners in no doubt that you know this by mentioning it early. You will need to assess them immediately and put out a crash call.

A–E

Airway

The patient is breathless and unable to speak, and I would be most concerned that this swelling represents a post-thyroidectomy haematoma compromising the airway. As such, I would ask the nurse to put out a 2222 call and also to contact the ENT registrar on call, as well as the anaesthetist on call, while I proceed to manage the patient.

I would sit the patient up and apply 15 L supplemental oxygen via a non-rebreather mask. I would enact the 'SCOOP' protocol – the kit for this should be at the bedside of the patient. This involves removing the steristrips and then cutting the subcuticular stitches of the anterior neck wound. I would then place my gloved fingers into the wound and open the skin to expose the strap muscles. The strap muscles are then opened to expose the trachea. In doing so, any accumulated haematoma will be evacuated. The wound is covered with a sterile wound pack. I would then reassess the airway and ensure that the patient has a patent and protected airway.

Further airway management would be led by the anaesthetist and the ENT registrar on call. The patient will need a return to theatre for haemostasis, and I would begin the workup for this. This would involve ensuring the patient had IV access, preoperative bloods were taken including a clotting and group and saves, and that I had spoken to the theatre coordinator, ENT and anaesthetics teams on call, as well as the ITU team to arrange a postoperative high-dependency bed. I would ensure the patient was nil by mouth, consented, and marked. In the meantime, I would consider giving the patient IV tranexamic acid to help reduce bleeding. I would ensure the patient is being very closely monitored for this period.

Breathing
- You would not move on to assess the breathing until you were completely satisfied that there was a stable, secure, patent airway; or that the anaesthetist was appropriately managing the airway and you were able to complete your assessment.

Circulation
- IV access and a VBG for a rapid assessment of their hgb, as well as FBC, clotting, and group and saves given postoperative bleeding. Examine any surgical drains to quantify additional bleeding.

Disability
- GCS or AVPU score is important to document with a mind to the patient's ability to maintain their own airway.

Exposure

AAPS

– Your senior should be involved immediately. Given the preceding events strong analgesia would be warranted.

History, Notes, Investigation

– The operation note should be reviewed. Any indication that the patient was at higher risk for postoperative complications should have been highlighted in the WHO sign-out. Check for documented intraoperative haemostasis issues.

Preliminary/Further Management

– As detailed above, a return to theatre is necessary – an urgent theatre workup required (see Section 9.2 for theatre workup). Postoperatively close monitoring of the patient is required.
– Whilst the patient is in theatre you could ensure the post-thyroidectomy emergency box was restocked and that other members of staff were adequately debriefed following what was likely a highly stressful episode.
– Once the patient is stabilised, make sure they are provided with suitable information about what has happened and what the plan is going forward – the episode may have been extremely distressing for them.

What might be contained within a post-thyroidectomy emergency box?
– SCOOP guideline
– Scissors and scalpel
– Gauze/ wound pack
– Artery clip
– Sterile gloves

What signs might aid early identification of this pathology
The acronym DESATS is useful here: Difficulty swallowing/discomfort; increase in Early warning score (EWS); Swelling; Anxiety; Tachypnoea/difficulty breathing; and Stridor.

What other complications of thyroid surgery should patients be consented for?
I would reference general complications such as pain, infection, bleeding/haematoma, seroma, scarring, and risks of a general anaesthetic. I would also reference risks specific to this operation including post-thyroidectomy haematoma, vocal cord palsy and voice change which may be temporary or permanent, the need for tracheostomy, hypothyroidism, and parathyroid gland injury requiring vitamin D and calcium support which may be temporary or permanent.

9.13 Postoperative Pyrexia

You are the on-call general surgical SHO. You are called by a nurse on the ward asking you to review a 59-year-old male complaining of severe abdominal pain. He is febrile at

38.4°C, his BP is 95/60 and his HR is 110. The patient is five days post resection of low rectal cancer with primary anastomosis. How would you approach this patient?

Before you begin: A classic scenario, and one that you would be foolish to not be well prepared for. A verbatim A–E approach is already written in the introductory chapter. The low rectal anastomosis is a clue that this is an anastomotic leak. This is a major class of postoperative complication; around a third of deaths after colorectal surgery are associated with anastomotic leaks.

A–E
Airway
Breathing
-   Start O_2 as part of the SEPSIS 6 bundle.

Circulation
-   Shocked patient to be managed as per CCRISP guidelines with large bore IV access in each ACF + full set of bloods including VBG + cultures, followed by crystalloid fluid resuscitation.
-   Response to fluid resuscitation should be closely monitored – transient responses which then fall again may indicate ongoing postoperative bleeding.
-   Catheterisation is essential for fluid balance monitoring.
-   ECG for tachycardia.

Disability
-   Temperature, GCS, and CBG are all essential here.

Exposure
-   Full abdominal examination including taking down dressings and examining wound.
-   Assess drains for faeculent output, pus or blood.

AAPS
-   Analgesia and early escalation to registrar.

History, Notes, Investigation
-   AMPLE history, pain history, and associated GI symptoms.
-   Chart review to assess op note and determine postoperative course including trends in observations.
-   Further investigation will likely be with CT abdo pelvis with IV contrast; however, this will vary based on the patient's stability – failure to improve with fluid resuscitation may warrant proceeding to urgent laparotomy if there is clinical suspicion of an intra-abdominal complication.

You perform a CT scan which demonstrates an anasomtotic leak; what are the management options?
Anastomotic leaks can be managed conservatively, medically, radiologically, and surgically. Conservative management involves keeping the patient NBM for bowel rest, insertion of an

NG tube to decompress the stomach, and IV fluid supplementation. Medical management involves the use of antibiotics – minor leaks may settle with this alone. Radiological management will involve the percutaneous drainage of larger intra-abdominal collections. Surgical management typically involves a washout and drainage of the contamination, followed by either resection of the anastomosis and creation of an end colostomy (Hartmann's procedure), and/or proximal faecal diversion with a defunctioning proximal stoma (ileostomy), with or without refashioning the anastomosis. Careful postoperative aftercare would be required, and may include total parenteral nutrition.

What risk factors predispose patients to having an anastomotic leak?
- Preoperative: smoking, diabetes, PVD, steroid use, poor nutritional state, anaemia, liver cirrhosis.
- Intraoperative: prolonged operative time, level of anastomosis, surgical technique to form anastomosis, tension on anastomosis, blood supply to anastomosis, and presence of contamination.
- Postoperative: infection, postoperative inflammatory states, poor nutrition due to reduced oral intake.

How do anastomotic leaks present?
The typical history is around day 5–7 following a low rectal anastomosis presenting with a peritonitic abdomen, severe abdominal pain, fever, and haemodynamic instability. It is important to note that it can present more vaguely, with vague abdominal pain, low-grade fever, prolonged postoperative ileus, low grade fever, or persistent tachycardia.

What is the POSSUM score?
The Physiological and Operative Severity Score for the enumeration of Mortality and morbidity, first developed in 1991, is used to predict morbidity and mortality for a wide range of surgical procedures. It measures both physiological parameters (e.g. a patient's age, their blood pressure, and bloods such as hgb and urea), as well as operative parameters (type of operation, NCEPOD classification, operative blood loss).

What is your differential for a postoperative fever in a patient who has undergone an abdominal operation?
A useful way to categorise differentials is by a (very rough) timeline of when different conditions may present:
- Day 1–2: infective causes which preceded the operation, such as CAP or UTI, reactions to anaesthetic agents, and the physiological response to surgery.
- Day 3–5: infective causes which followed the operation such as HAP, aspiration pneumonia, UTI, and surgical wound infections.
- Day 5–7: intra-abdominal pathology such as abscesses, collections, and anastomotic leaks.
- Anytime: transfusion and drug reactions, VTE, cardiac events, infected lines.

How is sepsis defined? How is septic shock defined?
Sepsis is defined as life-threatening organ dysfunction caused by a dysregulated host response to infection. Septic shock is defined as sepsis with associated circulatory (as well

as cellular and metabolic) abnormalities, which is associated with a greater mortality risk than sepsis alone.

9.14 Geriatric Fall

You are called to the emergency department to review an 89-year-old woman who was found at home after a fall. She is complaining of severe right groin pain and her right leg is shortened and externally rotated. She has a background of mild cognitive impairment, osteoporosis, and hypertension. How do you proceed?

Before you begin: Remember that this is a trauma patient – they may need a trauma call! Do not underestimate the dangers of a fall – they are the most common mechanism of fatal injury in the elderly population. A trauma call is the safest way to manage these 'silver trauma' patients and identify concurrent pathology. When going through your A–E, adding a choice few of the extra points listed below relating to geriatric trauma cases (*written in italics*) will help mark you out as a strong candidate. BOA have produced standards of care of the older or frail orthopaedic trauma patient, which you should familiarise yourself with [1]. It may be that in your scenario the patient has already had a trauma call assessment and been stabilised by ED.

A–E

C-Spine

- *Geriatric patients have more complications related to immobility (such as pressure sores and delirium) so early removal of cervical collars is used where possible. You cannot clinically clear the C-spine if the patient is uncooperative, as may be the case with an elderly delirious patient [2].*

Airway

- *Beware of dentures which can obstruct the airway, and arthritic changes which can make intubation more difficult.*

Breathing

- *Elderly patients are more likely to suffer rib fractures during falls which can impede breathing.*

Circulation

- Assess for signs of blood loss from bony fracture. Consider a pelvic binder if there are concerns about pelvic injury.
- Full set of bloods for geriatric assessment and preoperative workup including FBC, U&Es, VBG, clotting, group and saves, bone profile, and CK – patient may have had a long lie and be at risk of rhabdomyolysis.
- *Pre-existing hypertension may mask a relative hypotensive state. Elderly patients are also less able to increase HR to improve tissue perfusion, which may be worsened by beta-blocker use.*
- *Be vigilant to background use of anticoagulation/antiplatelet agents in this group which will worsen haemorrhage.*

Disability

- *Clearly record GCS in these patients at admission and have it regularly rechecked for deterioration. Assess for need for CT head as per NICE guidelines.*
- *The aging atrophied brain is more prone to traumatic brain injury.*
- *Decreased subcutaneous fat stores make hypothermia more likely.*

Exposure

- Full top-to-toe examination including logroll to identify other injuries before focusing on the affected area. Inspect for deformity, swelling, open wounds, discolouration, and bruising. Palpate for tenderness, distal neurovascular status, temperature, and haematoma. Move the joints of the lower limb and compare with other side. A fractured NOF will typically be shortened and externally rotated.

AAPS

- *Adjust analgesia doses to compensate for decreased liver/renal function.*
- Fascia iliaca block will provide good analgesia for a fractured NOF and is often part of local protocols for management of a fractured NOF.

History, Notes, Investigation

- History of the fall – clarify if there are medical concerns regarding the fall, such as a loss of consciousness, that will need workup. Determine if CT head will be needed as per NICE guidelines.
- Investigate the cause of the fall – ECG, CXR, urine dip, full blood panel including bone profile, recent medications, and compliance with medications should be determined.
- XRs: AP pelvis, cross table lateral, and full-length femoral view. If there is doubt about the diagnosis, then consider further imaging: MRI is the gold standard but CT is more readily available. N.B. the full-length femur views will help you identify skip lesions and therefore help with preoperative planning/management.
- AMTS/4AT assessment at baseline.

Preliminary Management

- Consider splinting with a foam gutter splint.
- Admit patient under joint care with geriatric team/frailty pathway as per 'Best practice tariff' guidance.
- Ensure early discussions about DNACPR and treatment escalation plans are had.
- Theatre workup including identifying and treating correctable co-morbidities.
- A catheter should be inserted for patients who are unlikely to be able to mobilise sufficiently to go to the toilet.

Further Management

- Benefits of surgical intervention will nearly always outweigh potential risk. Perform surgery on the day of or day after admission as per NICE guidance [3].

- Intracapsular fractures: management depends on the degree of displacement of the fracture (Garden classification). Nondisplaced fractures in young patients may be amenable to internal fixation, otherwise arthroplasty is required. Displaced fractures will need either hemiarthroplasty or total hip replacement (THR). NICE guidelines (2023) [3] recommend THR instead of hemiarthroplasty in patients who:
  - ○ Were able to walk independently out of doors with no more than the use of a stick AND
  - ○ Do not have a condition or comorbidity that makes the procedure unsuitable for them AND
  - ○ Are expected to be able to carry out activities of daily living independently beyond two years.
- Intertrochanteric fractures: consider dynamic hip screw
- Subtrochanteric and reverse oblique fractures: consider long intramedullary nail
- Postoperatively the patient should be managed with orthogeriatrics, aiming for early mobilisation on the day after arthroplasty surgery as per NICE guidance. Minimising bedbound time is key as elderly patients decondition quickly. Assessments of bone health, VTE risk, pressure sores, pain, nutrition, and delirium should be undertaken, as well as a comprehensive geriatric assessment with occupational therapy input.

What is the blood supply to the femoral head?

The main supply arises from the trochanteric anastomosis of the medial and lateral circumflex arteries and the superior gluteal artery, which run retrograde within the capsule. There is a small supply from ligamentum teres (artery of ligamentum teres) and from vessels with medullary canal.

What is the classification system for intracapsular NOF fractures?

The Garden classification categorises intracapsular NOF fractures by severity and degree of displacement:

I: Incomplete or valgus-impacted fracture.
II: Complete fracture which is undisplaced
III: Complete fracture with incomplete displacement (some continuity between fracture fragments).
IV: Complete fracture with complete displacement (no continuity between fracture fragments).

What risk factors do you know for NOF fractures?

Most risk factors relate to increasing osteoporosis risk. There are modifiable risk factors, such as steroid use, smoking, and low BMI. There are also non-modifiable risk factors such as advancing age, female gender, and worsening mobility. Comorbidities that make falling more likely include neuromuscular disorders like Parkinson's disease, visual and vestibular disorders, and dementia.

What complications should patients be aware of following an intracapsular NOF fracture managed with arthroplasty?
I would advise them about immediate, early, and late complications. Immediate complications include GA risks, cement reaction, perioperative fractures, and damage to nearby neurovascular structures (e.g. superior gluteal artery/nerve, sciatic nerve). Early complications include pain, VTE, surgical infections, hospital-acquired infections (chest, urine, etc.), and other medical complications (e.g. heart attacks/strokes), including risk of death. Late complications include leg length discrepancy, dislocation (around 10% rate with THR), periprosthetic fractures, delayed infection of metalwork, and aseptic loosening. N.B. in the case of internal fixation, the key complication is avascular necrosis of the femoral head, as well as non-union and infection of metalwork.

How is a fascia iliaca block placed?
A difficult question, but seeing as it is now considered part of the standard of care for a NOF fracture, it is worth knowing.

Ensure no contraindications (such as concurrent use of anticoagulant, local infection), and gain informed consent. A successful block will infiltrate local anaesthetic into the potential space under the fascia iliaca, blocking the femoral, lateral femoral cutaneous, and obturator nerves. This can be performed using a landmark technique or under ultrasound guideline. Find the ASIS and pubic tubercle, find the junction between the lateral one-third and medial two-third between these two structures, and go 1–2 cm distal to this point. Identify the femoral artery and ensure your insertion point is lateral to this (the nerve lies lateral to the artery). Under ultrasound guidance, or using the landmark technique, the needle is inserted, feeling for the two 'pops' as the needle passes through fascia lata and then the fascia iliaca. Aspirate to ensure you are not in a vessel, then inject 1–2 ml local anaesthetic (levobupivacaine is often used, maximum dose 2 mg/kg) to confirm needle placement – under ultrasound the fascia should be seen to separate from the iliacus if correctly positioned. Complete injection with remaining volume of local anaesthetic, aspirating every 5 ml. Monitor the patient for 30 minutes afterwards, looking for signs of LA toxicity.

References

1. BOA (n.d.). 'BOAST – The care of the older or frail orthopaedic trauma patient'. Website, www.boa.ac.uk, accessed 19 Feb. 2024, www.boa.ac.uk/resource/boast-frailty.html.

2. BOA (n.d.). 'BOAST – Cervical spine clearance in the trauma patient'. Website, www.boa.ac.uk, accessed 19 Feb. 2024, www.boa.ac.uk/resource/boast-cervical-spine-clearance-in-the-trauma-patient.html.

3. NICE (n.d.). 'Hip fracture: Management'. Website, accessed 19 Feb. 2024, www.nice.org.uk/guidance/cg124/chapter/Recommendations#surgical-procedures. Reproduced with permission.

9.15 Pelvic Trauma

You are the orthopaedic CT1 bleeped to resus where a 19-year-old man has been brought in by ambulance following a head-on road traffic collision at 60 mph. He is complaining of groin pain and the ambulance crew noted blood visible at the urethral meatus. He is tachycardic at 110, BP 100/70, RR 19, Sats 98% on room air. How do you proceed?

Before you begin: Ensure a trauma call has been put out and your senior is aware of the patient. This is a high-energy mechanism of injury in a young patient who is haemodynamically unstable. There are several things that may be causing this, but the mechanisms of injury with groin pain and blood at the urethral meatus should make you concerned about pelvic injuries and genitourinary trauma – these injuries often present simultaneously. Haematuria in trauma should make you concerned about renal, ureteric, bladder, or urethral injuries, but remember that management of the haemodynamic compromise is the first priority. BOA standards exist for the management of both pelvic trauma [1] and associated urological injury [2]. There is a lot to say in the workup of this scenario, which makes covering everything difficult. Remember that providing a comprehensive overview of the workup is more important than knowing specific details around genitourinary trauma.

A–E
C-Spine
Airway
Breathing
– Although respiratory observations are normal, you should be providing a comprehensive trauma A–E in this situation given the high-energy mechanism.

Circulation
– Tachycardia and hypotension here is haemorrhage until proven otherwise. Search for source of haemorrhage ('on the floor and four more') with an eFAST scan as required. Gently palpate the pelvis for instability – do not 'spring' the pelvis as this may distract the fracture, dislodging clots and causing further bleeding.
– Apply a pelvic binder: hypotensive patients with a history of pelvic trauma should be assumed to have a pelvic fracture until proven otherwise.
– Activate major haemorrhage protocol.
– Large bore cannula in each ACF. One litre bolus of warmed IV crystalloid, and titrate further fluids to response, reassessing from 'airway' after each intervention, and replacing 'like for like' with packed RBC as soon as possible. Full set of bloods including FBC, U&Es, LFTs, two group and saves (with urgent cross match), and bone profile for preoperative workup. VBG to check lactate and for a rapid assessment of hgb.
– IV TXA within one hour.
– Consider catheterisation – in the context of possible urethral damage this should be done in consultation with urology (see below).

N.B. in your interview you should state that you should not move on from 'C' until the patient is haemodynamically stable, and bleeding is controlled. However, you can explain that while fluid resuscitation is ongoing and you are monitoring the response to this, you would continue your assessment.

Disability

– Ensure adequate patient warming in major haemorrhage situations (e.g. Bair hugger). Hypothermia is one component of the trauma triad of death.

Exposure

– Complete a full top-to-toe examination including log roll.
– Examination of pelvis and lower limbs looking for pain, swelling, deformity, and leg length discrepancy. Distal neurovascular assessment must be performed.
– Examination of genitals and perineum looking for blood at the urethral meatus, bruising or haematoma of scrotum of perineum.
– PR – prostate may be boggy or displaced in urethral injuries. Bony fragments present in the rectum would reclassify this as an 'open fracture' in terms of your management, and general surgery input will be needed.

AAPS

– Senior review is essential here, and having the correct expertise is worth mentioning – pelvic fractures of this nature should be managed at major trauma centres, orthopaedics and urology should be present, and given how unwell the patient is, critical care/ITU outreach should be contacted. Interventional radiology services can be involved for consideration of embolisation of bleeding pelvic vessels. Theatres should be aware of the patient early and workup performed (Section 9.2).

History, Notes, Investigations

– AMPLE history, determining the vector of force and speed of both cars, is important.
– As per BOA standards, patients with suspected pelvic fracture should have a trauma CT 'panscan' with contrast [1].
– After discussion with urology, the patient may need a retrograde urethrogram.

Preliminary and Definitive Management

– Aggressive resuscitation as detailed above.
– If there is urine leak from the bladder or urethra, or signs of bony fragments in the rectum, then pelvic fracture must be treated like an open fracture.
– Haemorrhage secondary to pelvic fracture can be controlled with angiographic embolisation or surgical packing of the pelvis. Fracture management depends on degree of instability and displacement, but external fixation may be used to temporarily stabilise the pelvis prior to definitive surgery being performed; pelvic reconstruction should occur within 72 hours if the patient is stabilised [1].
– Urological input for bladder and urethral injuries (see below).

How do you apply a pelvic binder?
Internally rotate the patient's legs at the hip, and then apply the binder at the level of the greater trochanters, tighten it, and secure it. It should not be used for more than 24 hours due to risk of ulceration over bony prominences. Be particularly careful in men as

genitalia can become trapped within the binder and lead to ischaemia. An XR should always be performed following removal of a pelvic binder even in the presence of a 'normal' CT scan as applying the binder may be masking pelvic disruption on imaging.

What classification exists for pelvic fractures?

The Young and Burgess classification [3] is based on the vector of force causing the fracture – different directions of force result in different patterns of injuries to the pelvic ring. This includes anterior–posterior compression, lateral compression, and vertical shear fractures.

Should you catheterise in suspected urethral trauma?

BOA standards advise a single, gentle attempt at catheterisation by an experienced doctor even in the presence of clinical or radiological evidence of urethral injury [2]. If frank blood is present or the catheter is not passing then stop and withdraw, a suprapubic catheter will be needed. Note that the latest edition of ATLS (10th edition, 2018) states that transurethral bladder catheterisation is contraindicated for patients who may have urethral injury and a retrograde urethrogram is mandatory in these situations [4]. Urology input should be sought if there are concerns.

How is a retrograde urethrogram performed?

XR plate is placed under the pelvis. A small foley catheter balloon within the meatus is gently inflated and 20 ml of dilute contrast dye is injected through it. Lateral and AP pelvic XRs are taken to observe for contrast leak.

How do you examine the urological system in pelvic trauma?

In addition to the abdominal exam and pelvic exam (a single check for pelvic instability before applying the binder), examine the perineum and external genitalia. You should look for any signs of haemorrhage, bruising, and deformity. A PR exam should be conducted to check for a displaced prostate, loss of anal canal integrity, or sharp bony objects. If there are signs of a bony fracture penetrating the anal canal, this should be treated as an open fracture.

How do you manage urethral injury in trauma?

Typically, this does not require primary repair – the urethra is easily damaged in the hands of less experienced surgeons – and is instead repaired at around three months, but urology input should be sought. All patients should be counselled on potential urinary sexual dysfunction after management.

How do you manage bladder injury in trauma?

The key distinction is whether it is intraperitoneal or extraperitoneal. If intraperitoneal, an emergency laparotomy is typically needed. Extraperitoneal can often be managed conservatively with catheterisation.

What types of catheters do you know?

- Straight tip
- Curved tip Coude tip/Tiemann tip
- Three-way catheter for continuous bladder irrigation

- Suprapubic catheter
- Open tip catheter
- Condom/sheath/external catheter

References

1. BOA (n.d.). 'BOAST – The management of patients with pelvic fractures'. Website, www.boa.ac.uk, www.boa.ac.uk/resource/boast-3-pdf.html.

2. BOA (n.d.). 'BOAST – The management of urological trauma associated with pelvic fractures'. Website, www.boa.ac.uk, accessed 19 Feb. 2024, www.boa.ac.uk/resource/boast-14-pdf.html.

3. Young JW, Burgess AR, Brumback RJ, Poka A (1986). 'Pelvic fractures: Value of plain radiography in early assessment and management'. *Radiology* 160(2): 445–451, https://doi.org/10.1148/radiology.160.2.3726125.

4. American College of Surgeons (2018). *Committee on Trauma. ATLS: Student Course Manual*. Chicago, Ill.: American College of Surgeons.

9.16 Neck Lump

You are the ENT CT1 on call and are asked to come to the urgent care centre to assess a 26-year-old man with a large, rapidly growing neck lump in the midline, around the region of his tracheal cartilage. The patient is clinically well, speaking normally, and not in pain. Observations are stable. Routine blood tests are normal. How do you proceed?

Before you begin: This is a patient with a stable presentation and the A–E assessment should therefore be brief. A thorough neck examination and a strong differential are more important in this station.

A–E

This patient appears well. I would assess the patient with a CCRISP-guided A–E approach to ensure the patient is stable, with particular focus on ensuring this lump did not obstruct or threaten the airway. If there are any aberrations in my A–E assessment, I would treat them before continuing. I would then proceed to a focused history and examination of the neck.

History and Examination

I would take a thorough history from the patient. This would include demographic details, a structured history of the lump including the time of onset, any precipitating factors, and the speed of growth. I would enquire about associated red flag symptoms involving the upper aero-digestive tract, such as pain, dysphonia, dysphagia, odynophagia, referred otalgia, unilateral nasal obstruction, and unilateral hearing loss. Given this is a midline lump I would also enquire about symptoms of hyperthyroidism and hypothyroidism. I would ask about a history of previous lumps, and their medical/drug/social history. I would assess for risk factors for carcinoma such as prior radiation exposure (for papillary thyroid cancer) or history of other cancers (such as parathyroid carcinoma and phaeochromocytomas associated with MEN 2A).

To examine the lump, I would take an inspect, palpate, percuss, auscultate approach. I would inspect for the site, size, and surrounding skin changes, as well as how the lump moves when swallowing and on tongue protrusion. I would palpate the lump for consistency, mobility, tenderness, temperature, transillumination, and its relation to nearby structures, as well as the presence of lymphadenopathy. I would percuss for retrosternal extension and auscultate for bruits. I would also examine for stigmata of thyroid disease and assess the character of the patient's voice.

N.B. you may not have time to cover every element of the neck examination. By smoothly and fluently covering the highlights and bits relevant to this presentation, you are highlighting an understanding of the necessary approach.

Ongoing Assessment

Following the examination, I would organise radiological and cytological characterisation of the lesion, which can usually be achieved with ultrasound + FNA, to complete the 'triple assessment' of the lump. The remainder of my assessment would be guided by my findings. This may involve a full thyroid examination, examination of the oral/nasal cavity, flexible nasendoscopy, and blood tests, including TFTs.

Outline the Differential for This Neck Lump

This can be categorised in many ways (e.g. into midline vs lateral, anatomical triangles, or a surgical sieve). Examiners want to know that you understand the specific differentials for this scenario (a midline lump), and that you can structure differentials logically.

Given the midline location and proximity to the tracheal cartilage, the most likely differentials in this case include thyroid causes such as goitre, thyroid nodule, thyroid cancer, or thyroglossal duct cyst, an non-thyroid causes such as lymphadenopathy, midline branchial cysts, dermoid cysts, and vascular malformations.

The FNA results indicate the patient has a papillary thyroid cancer. What is the management?

As with all cancer diagnoses, a patient-centred holistic approach should be used through an MDT setting. The diagnosis should be explained to the patient, and the patient supported with this news as required. Further staging investigations may be performed such as CT to establish the TNM status of the disease. Management options include a watch-and-wait surveillance approach, thyroid lobectomy, and total thyroidectomy with or without dissection of the surrounding lymph nodes. Following surgical management, some patients will receive radioiodine to ablate residual thyroid tissue. The management pathway chosen will depend on the specific grade and stage of the tumour, the patient's desires and expectations, and the patient's fitness for intervention.

9.17 Postoperative Confusion

You are the general surgical CT1. An 82-year-old patient has become increasingly confused on day 1 after a Hartmann's procedure for bowel cancer. There is no documented history of underlying cognitive impairment. The nurse is concerned and has called to ask you for help. Observations: HR 78, BP 160/85, RR 18, Sats 94% on RA, apyrexial. Please outline your approach to this patient.

Before you begin: In this case you want to demonstrate a strong differential (see below) for postoperative confusion (precipitating causes) whilst acknowledging that there are predisposing factors to be aware of. While postoperative delirium is common, saying this as a diagnosis alone is insufficient – you must understand how to assess for underlying causes.

A–E
Airway
Breathing
- Oxygen saturations should be rechecked as hypoxia is a potential cause of delirium.
- Auscultate the chest to check for basal crackles.

Circulation
- When sending bloods, ensure you send a full confusion screen including U&Es to check electrolytes, FBC and CRP, bone profile, thyroid function tests, and LFTs.

Disability
- A GCS, temperature and capillary blood glucose are all essential.
- A gross neurological exam to check for focal neurology which may indicate potential cerebrovascular accident (CVA).

Exposure
- Check any indwelling lines, and if the patient has a catheter ensure it is draining.
- A full abdominal exam, including checking the wound site and for signs of peritonism.
- A fluid status exam, ensuring the nursing staff are monitoring and recording urine output accurately.

AAPS
- Ensure the patient has adequate analgesia, as pain can cause delirium.
- Inform the operating surgeon or on-call registrar.

History, Notes, Investigation
- Cognitive screening test such as AMTS, CAM, or 4AT scoring.
- Take a collateral history from the nursing staff looking after the patient. Check for any predisposing factors, including sensory impairment, recent environmental changes, poor sleep as per nursing notes, dehydration or malnutrition. When time allows, a comprehensive collateral history from the NOK will be essential to determine the cognitive baseline for the patient – just because there is no cognitive impairment documented does not necessarily mean that this is really the case.
- Review the notes for previous episodes of delirium, comorbidities, and the operative note for blood loss. Check stool charts.
- Review patient's medications for predisposing agents such as opioids, anticholinergics, antihistamines, and steroids. Also, check for any missed

medications such as VTE prophylaxis, antibiotics, or neurological agents such as Parkinson's medications.
- Send bloods (as above) including a VBG, send urine dip/MC&S and wound swabs, and consider an ECG, CXR, and CT head, based on clinical findings.

Preliminary Management
- The management will depend on the underlying cause of the confusion; however, it's worth being aware of measures that can generally help to reduce delirium in patients. For example: minimising polypharmacy, ensuring pain is well controlled, hydration and nutrition are optimised, and sleep disruption is minimised.
- Delirium is associated with prolonged hospital stays and increased mortality. Perform a thorough workup and get a medical review.

What is the differential for the causes of postoperative delirium?
- Infection: including HAP, COVID, wound, lines, catheters, abscess, collection.
- Respiratory: hypoxia, hypercarbia.
- Drugs: analgesia, sedatives.
- Electrolyte abnormalities: hyponatraemia from excessive IV filling, SIADH, perioperative glucose derangement.
- Cerebrovascular event such as stroke.
- Other: dehydration, malnutrition, sleep deprivation, moving wards, constipation, pain.

What are the predisposing factors for postoperative delirium?
Preoperative factors include:
- Reduced cognitive reserve due to age or cognitive impairment.
- Reduced physical reserve due to comorbidities such as cardiovascular disease and renal impairment, sarcopenia.
- Pre-existing sensory impairment.
- Malnutrition.

Intraoperative factors include:
- Use of a general anaesthetic, prolonged operative time, substantial physiological insult (major surgery), substantial blood loss.

Postoperative factors include:
- Missed medications.
- Sleep deprivation.
- Changing environment and overstimulation.
- Pain.

What is the definition of delirium?
An acute, reversible, transient period of fluctuating consciousness, reduced alertness, and inattention. It is an acute confusional state.

The patient is confused, and is trying to leave the ward, adamant that she 'needs to get to Buckingham Palace as she has an important meeting to attend'. How do you proceed?

The patient should be gently talked to and encouraged to come back to her bedside for a discussion about why it's important she stays. Involving the family so the patient has recognisable faces may be helpful. If all available reasoning options fail, and a patient who has been shown to lack capacity is persistently trying to leave when it is clearly unsafe for them to do so, then it is necessary to prevent them from leaving. This will require the completion of a DoLS (Deprivation of Liberty Safeguards). This is the legal procedure used to protect the rights of individuals who lack capacity in these situations, ensuring that any limitation in the patient's liberty is appropriate and in their best interests.

9.18 Vomiting Child

You are the general surgical CT1. You are bleeped by the paediatric emergency department to review a five-week-old boy who has persistent non-bilious projectile vomiting. The boy feeds enthusiastically after vomiting but vomits again soon afterwards. How do you proceed?

Before you begin: A vomiting five-week-old child could have multiple aetiologies, including simple gastroenteritis, gastro-oesophageal reflux, urinary tract infection, or food allergy. However, the age range (three to six weeks), gender, projectile nature of the vomit with enthusiastic post-vomit feeding (and most importantly the fact that this is a surgical interview!), should point you in the direction of pyloric stenosis.

N.B. paediatric scenarios are less likely, but if they do arise, your primary focus is to appear a safe trainee who acts within their competence. Early senior support and paediatric input should be sought for all unwell children. However, having a strong understanding of paediatric fluid prescribing is useful clinically, and will mark you out as a good candidate.

A–E

Airway

- If vomitus is obstructing the airway, clear the airway with suctioning and positioning.

Breathing
Circulation

- Assess the child's hydration status, looking to differentiate clinical dehydration (around 5% fluid loss) from clinical shock (around 10% fluid loss). N.B. NICE have produced a useful guide for assessing this [1].

While examining the unwell child for signs of clinical dehydration, I would first look generally, for irritability, lethargy, and an unwell appearance. On closer examination I would assess for sunken eyes, sunken fontanelles, dry mucous membranes, and reduced skin turgor. I would look for tachycardia, normotension, and reduced urine output. I would be concerned this had progressed to clinical shock (10% loss) if I noted decreased consciousness, pale or mottled skin, a prolonged capillary refill time or hypotension. Seeing signs of shock should warrant putting out a paediatric crash call to ensure appropriate expertise was on hand to help manage this case.

I would commence fluid balance charts including monitoring urine output. Given this patient is not tolerating oral feeding, it is likely that IV supplementation will be required. When IV access is being placed, I would request that a full set of bloods were taken with a mind to potential operative management. This would also include a VBG – the lactate is a marker of shock, and the VBG typically demonstrates hypochloraemic hypokalaemic metabolic alkalosis in pyloric stenosis.

For shock, with paediatric supervision, as per NICE guidance, glucose-free crystalloids with sodium in the range 131–154 mmol/L should be used, beginning with 10 ml/kg over 10 minutes [2]. Up to three 10 ml/kg boluses after which urgent expert advice from paediatrics/PICU is needed as inotropes should be considered. I would ask about underlying cardiac disease and renal disease before giving fluid boluses. Once resuscitated, fluid deficit and daily fluid maintenance requirements should be calculated and provided.

Disability
- Use paediatric GCS.

Exposure
- Full abdominal assessment looking for signs of pyloric stenosis such as olive-shaped mass (this is the hypertrophied pyloric muscle) found inferior to the liver edge and visible peristalsis from left to right (as the stomach attempts to force food across the stenosed outlet).

AAPS
- As mentioned above, early senior input should be sought.

History, Notes, Investigation
- Ask about feeding (breast feeding: how many minutes per breast, and how often, bottles: expressed breast milk or formula, how many ml per bottle, and how often) and wet nappies (<2 in 12 hours is concerning). Ask about formula changes – note that stenosis can present with vague symptoms sometimes mistaken for intolerance of different types of formula.
- Growth and development history. See red book and check weights since birth – plot all weights on an age- and gender-appropriate growth chart – they may be failing to grow, or dropping centiles.
- Immunisations and past medical history.
- Risk factors for pyloric stenosis: Western heritage, family history, first born child, and male.
- Ultrasound is most commonly used – pylorus muscle thickness >3–5 mm and pyloric canal length >15 mm are the diagnostic thresholds for full-term infants.

Preliminary Management
- Continue fluid resuscitation, make the child NBM, pass a nasogastric tube to decompress the stomach and commence theatre workup.
- Consider a test feed (dummy dipped in breast milk or infant formula) to aid diagnosis after gastric tube has been passed.

Further Management

- Ramstedt's pyloromyotomy is most commonly performed after correction of the metabolic alkalosis – the pyloric muscle is split longitudinally. This can be performed open or laparoscopically.
- Reassure the parent/caregiver as this is likely a highly stressful time for them. Note the success of surgical treatment nears 100% with very few complications.
- Infants are restarted on feeding once they have recovered from the anaesthesia.

How do you calculate the fluid deficit in clinical dehydration? How do you calculate maintenance requirements for a child?
Fluid deficit can be calculated by subtracting the child's current weight from a recent weight before the episode started. This weight difference in grams = fluid lost in millilitres. If there is no recent weight, then the equation is listed below:

> **Current weight × 10 × replacement percentage**
>
> *Note the replacement percentage in a clinically dehydrated patient is taken to be 5% (and 10% in a shocked child) e.g. in a clinically dehydrated child weighing 5 kg: 5 kg × 10 × 5 (%) = 250 ml. This is replaced over 24 hours, so the 5 kg child would need 250 ml each day on top of maintenance requirements.*

Maintenance fluid requirements are determined by weight: 100 ml/kg for the first 10 kg body weight, 50 ml/kg for the second 10 kg bodyweight, and 20 ml/kg for every kg above 20 kg bodyweight. Maintenance fluid is often given as 5% glucose with 0.9% sodium chloride, with an added 10 mmol KCl per 500 ml bag.

Why do these patients have their typical VBG findings?
Repeated vomiting leads to loss of hydrochloric acid, and a subsequent hypochloraemic metabolic alkalosis. In an attempt to conserve hydrogen ions, the kidneys retain hydrogen ions in exchange for potassium ions. This leads to a drop in potassium levels, hence the hypokalaemic hypochloraemic metabolic alkalosis.

What would you be most concerned about if the child was one month old presenting with bilious vomiting and abdominal discomfort?
The most concerning differential for bilious vomiting in this age group is malrotation with midgut volvulus. This occurs due to abnormal intestinal fixation, allowing the small bowel to rotate on its mesentery, obstructing the duodenum (hence bilious vomiting is seen). This can cause ischaemia and severe abdominal pain resulting in an inconsolable child. The abdomen is initially scaphoid, with distension and discolouration suggesting progression to gangrene of the twisted midgut. It is common practise to order an upper GI contrast series, looking for the position of the duodeno-jejunal junction. If this is displaced inferiorly, in the midline, or to the right of the midline, an urgent laparotomy is indicated to detort the midgut and divide Ladd's bands (fibres attaching the caecum to the retroperitoneum). An ultrasound can also be helpful to assess the relative positions of the SMA and SMV.

References

1. NICE (2009). 'Diarrhoea and vomiting caused by gastroenteritis in under 5s: Diagnosis and management | Guidance | NICE'. Website, Nice.org.uk, www.nice .org.uk/Guidance/CG84.

2. NICE (2015). 'Recommendations | Intravenous fluid therapy in children and young people in hospital | Guidance | NICE'. Website, Nice.org.uk, www.nice .org.uk/guidance/ng29/chapter/ Recommendations.

9.19 Haematemesis

You are called to the Emergency Department to assess a 64-year-old man who has presented with epigastric pain and haematemesis. His past medical history is notable for Cushing's disease for which he is on long-term steroid supplementation. Observations: HR 121, BP 95/65, RR 28, Sats 96% on RA. How would you proceed?

Before you begin: This patient is clearly extremely unwell with signs pointing to stage III shock – manage them in resus. The history of steroid use makes a bleeding peptic ulcer (a common cause of upper GI bleeding) the most likely differential. However, haematemesis has a wide differential, which we would classify anatomically. You can mention these now or at the end of your A–E to show that you are not jumping to conclusions – note that the initial workup for an UGIB will be similar for all of these.

Upper G.I. bleed differential
– Oesophagus: variceal bleed, oesophagitis, Mallory Weiss tear, tumour, Boerhaave's perforation.
– Stomach: gastric ulcers, tumour, Dieulafoy lesion (most commonly in gastric region).
– Duodenum: duodenal ulcers, duodenitis, aorto-duodenal fistula.
– SB: tumour, Meckel's, aortoenteric fistula, angiodysplasia.
– General: bleeding diathesis, hereditary haemorrhagic telangiectasia.

A–E

Airway

– Vomitus and blood can block airway – roll patient onto side and use suction where needed.

Breathing

– Aspiration following haematemesis can cause a drop in saturations.

Circulation

– Patient is in stage III shock and requires immediate resuscitation.
– Large bore IV access in each ACF and replace 'like for like' with RBC transfusion as early as possible, activation of the major haemorrhage protocol, and early haematology input regarding need for platelets and FFP.
– Full set of bloods with VBG (rapid hgb and lactate), clotting (coagulopathy), group and saves, with urgent cross matching. Thromboelastography (TEG) can be used as a rapid test to identify clotting abnormalities (if available).

- Catheterise to monitor fluid balance.
- ECG given tachycardia.

Disability
- Document GCS – confusion is a worrying sign of worsening shock.
- Monitor temperature closely.

Exposure
- Full abdominal assessment looking for signs pointing to aetiology, for example chronic liver disease (spider naevi, ascites, gynaecomastia). Perform PR exam (melaena).

AAPS
- This shocked patient must be escalated urgently to the general surgical registrar, gastroenterology, theatre teams, anaesthetics, and critical care outreach teams.

History, Notes, Investigation
- If able, AMPLE history. Identifying risk factors for peptic ulcers or other causes of UGI bleed, as well as a coagulation history, would be useful but is likely unrealistic given how unwell the patient is.
- Erect CXR (pneumomediastinum e.g. Boerhaave's, or pneumoperitoneum e.g. perforated ulcer). A lateral decubitus film can also be taken to assess for air between the liver and lateral abdominal wall. XR has the important advantage of being portable. CT with IV contrast is more sensitive if there are concerns about GI perforation but should only be performed when stable enough to be transferred to the radiology department. Some patients may proceed straight to endoscopy.

Preliminary Management
- Based on response to resuscitation, endoscopy may be required urgently – this is both diagnostic and therapeutic. Make NBM and prep for theatre (see Section 9.2). You can give erythromycin as a prokinetic to increase vision during endoscopy.
- Current NICE guidelines recommend PPI should not be given before endoscopy in suspected non-variceal bleeding and should only be given after endoscopy if there are stigmata of recent haemorrhage on OGD [1].
- If OGD is inconclusive, consider CT angiogram (useful in patients who are actively bleeding) and colonoscopy.
- Reversal of coagulation defects.

Further Management (of Peptic Ulcer)
- At endoscopy you can perform clipping + adrenaline injection, thermal coagulation + adrenaline injection, or fibrin/thrombin injection + adrenaline injection. Post-endoscopy Rockall score should be calculated.
- If this fails to stop the bleeding, consider repeat OGD, or angiographic embolisation (if interventional radiology is available).

– If this fails, or is not available, then the unstable patient should proceed to surgery – this may entail oversewing a bleeding gastroduodenal artery in the posterior duodenum or partial gastrectomy and drainage into a Roux-en-Y loop of jejunum

What scoring systems are used in upper GI bleeds?
While most will have heard of the Glasgow Blatchford and Rockall scores, stand out by knowing what exactly scoring systems are validated for. The Glasgow Blatchford score is used to determine which UGIBs are 'high risk' for requiring transfusions, endoscopy, or surgery. 'Low risk' bleeds (scoring 0) are safe for early discharge and outpatient management. The Rockall score is used after endoscopy to quantify both the risk of rebleeding and of overall mortality. This uses patient's Age, Blood pressure and heart rate, Comorbidities, Diagnosis at endoscopy, and Stigmata of recent haemorrhage at endoscopy (remembered as ABCDS).

How would your management change if the patient had a history of chronic alcohol use and known liver cirrhosis?
This would make a variceal bleed more likely. While typically seen as a 'medical' pathology, the basics of management are resuscitation, followed by terlipressin, prophylactic antibiotics, and endoscopic management (band ligation for oesophageal varices, N-butyl-2-cyanoacrylate injections for gastric varices). If this fails to control the bleeding, transjugular intrahepatic portosystemic shunts (TIPS) ± Sengstaken tube can be considered. Emergency surgery to form a vascular shunt is the last resort – it has a high mortality rate. Propranolol and consideration of repeat banding should be given after the interventions.

Reference

1. NICE (n.d.). 'Acute upper gastrointestinal bleeding in over 16s: Management | Guidance | NICE'.

Website, www.nice.org.uk, www.nice.org.uk/guidance/cg141/chapter/Recommendations#management-of-non-variceal-bleeding.

9.20 Fall from a Height

You are the general surgical SHO on call and are called to assess a 32-year-old female in resus who complains of left thigh pain and swelling after falling 3 m off a ladder. They are alert and their observations are stable. Please outline your approach to this patient.

Before you begin: Remember *life before limb*. Trauma cases require a full ATLS A–E approach, and immediately focusing on the limb may miss other, more life-threatening, injuries. A full ATLS A–E + full examination of an injured limb takes a long time – practise going through the whole case and practise examiners interrupting you to skip straight to examining the injured limb.

A–E

C-Spine

– Triple immobilisation of the C-spine with collar until the C-spine is cleared with blocks and tape is your first priority given the mechanism of injury.

Airway
Breathing
Circulation

- Swelling in the thigh may constitute a haematoma following femoral fracture. The femur is highly vascularised, and being vigilant for signs of circulatory compromise is key.
- The thigh compartment is one of the five areas of haemorrhage accumulation (chest, abdomen, pelvis, long bones, 'floor'/external). Swelling in the thigh may constitute haematoma, and the highly vascularised nature of the femur should mean you are vigilant for the signs of circulatory compromise – activating the major haemorrhage protocol is needed if there are concerns. Large bore IV access in each ACF with a full set of bloods including VBG, FBC, group and saves, and clotting is essential given the potential of a major bleed or the need to proceed to theatre.

Disability
Exposure

- Perform a full top-to-toe examination with log roll to identify concomitant life-threatening pathology followed by a comprehensive examination of the affected leg using a look, feel, move approach (see Section 9.8) with clear documentation of the neurovascular status of the limb.

AAPS

- Strong analgesia and a pregnancy test are essential, as is senior input.

History, Notes, Investigations

- AMPLE history, including confirming the height she fell from and the circumstances of the fall.
- Orthogonal view radiographs of affected area, the joint above and below (AP and lateral views) ± further imaging as indicated in the top-to-toe assessment. Given a possible femoral injury, it is important that imaging excludes injuries to the pelvis and femoral neck/head. Given the mechanism of injury a CT pan scan to include the femur would be performed.
- Note that as per Canadian C-spine rules, this patient has had a dangerous mechanism of injury which mandates radiological clearance of the C-spine.

What is the management of femoral midshaft fracture?

Detailed management on how to manage different fractures is unlikely to be needed (the exception to this may be NOFs), but having a clear structure is key:

As with all fractures I would take a reduce, hold, rehabilitate approach to managing this patient. Following the ATLS assessment I would ensure adequate analgesia is provided. Immediate reduction and immobilisation to near anatomic alignment using in-line traction should be performed – for example, with skin traction. Reducing the fracture will help manage the bleeding and pain. I would reassess neurovascular status after reduction.

Definitive management then typically occurs within 24–48 hours with plate fixation or intramedullary femoral nailing. As for many trauma fractures, if the fracture is unstable/open/part of polytrauma, then external fixation may be considered. Finally, the patient should undergo early mobilisation and intensive physiotherapy (as tolerated) to rehabilitate, reduce complication rates, and restore function of the limb.

What are the complications of a femoral midshaft fracture?

Stand out by ensuring you have a structure which allows you to answer confidently, even if not comprehensively. Again, you must categorise:

I would categorise the complications into immediate, early, and late complications. Immediate complications include haemorrhage and neurological injury. Early complications include fat embolism, compartment syndrome, VTE, and infection. Late complications include non-union, malunion, and weakness.

The patient has fallen from a height of 3 m. Can you clinically clear their C-spine without imaging?

Given this is a dangerous mechanism of injury, the C-spine requires radiological imaging to clear.

How could you 'clear' a C-spine in a trauma patient?

I would follow the BOA guidance on C-spine clearance in trauma [1]. This outlines the two ways you can clear a C-spine, either normal clinical examination in an awake and orientated patient or completion of spinal imaging protocols in all other patients for whom this is not suitable or there is suspicion of injury. Radiological imaging should follow local protocols, but in trauma scenarios may involve a trauma CT scan that includes the C-spine.

How might you clinically clear a C-spine without imaging?

To clinically clear the C-spine without any imaging, the Canadian C-spine rules can be used. First, I would ensure the patient had no 'high risk' factors which mandate radiological clearance (age ≥65, dangerous mechanism of injury, paraesthesia in upper or lower limbs). I would then confirm that the patient had at least one 'low risk' factor present (comfortable in a sitting position, ambulatory at any time since the accident, delayed and not immediate onset neck pain, no midline tenderness, and simple rear end motor vehicle collision as the mechanism of injury). If one of these 'low risk' factors was present I would remove triple immobilisation and ask the patient to rotate their neck 45 degrees in both directions – if they can, then the C spine is cleared.

Reference

1. BOA (n.d.). 'BOAST – Cervical spine clearance in the trauma patient'. Website, www.boa.ac.uk, https://www.boa.ac.uk/resource/boast-cervical-spine-clearance-in-the-trauma-patient.html.

9.21 Painful Leg Following Trauma

You are the orthopaedic CT1 called to the inpatient ward to review a 22-year-old male patient who came off his motorbike yesterday, suffering a closed fracture of his right tibial plateau and fibula. His lower leg was put in a circumferential plaster, and he is due a definitive operation to manage this on the trauma list tomorrow. He is now complaining of severe right lower leg pain. He is tachycardic at 110, but otherwise his observations are normal. How do you proceed?

Before you begin: This history is concerning for compartment syndrome, which is an orthopaedic emergency. The differential also includes inadequately controlled fracture-related pain or acutely ischaemic limbs and DVT, both of which are also potential emergencies. Stress the urgency of the situation and review them immediately. Stand out in this scenario by knowing (and referencing) the relevant BOA standards.

A–E

Airway

Breathing

- High-flow O_2 to improve O_2 delivery to potentially ischaemic tissues.

Circulation

- BOA standards advise maintaining a normal BP [1].
- IV fluids here may transiently improve perfusion of the limb – and may help bring heart rate down if his tachycardia is caused by dehydration (it may be elevated due to severe pain). Sufficient IV hydration for adequate urine output is also important in preventing kidney injury secondary to rhabdomyolysis.
- Catheterise to monitor UO and perform an ECG as tachycardic.
- Wide bore IV access. Bloods with a mind to potential operative management, and to monitor his CK.

Disability

Exposure

- Examination of the affected area with a look, feel, move approach, looking for key signs of compartment syndrome (see below). Severe pain alone is sufficient to raise suspicion. Paraesthesia, a pulseless limb, pallor, paralysis, and a 'perishingly cold' limb are all late signs which are associated with ischemia and therefore poor outcome – compartment syndrome should be picked up before these signs manifest.

Signs and symptoms of compartment syndrome

- Compartment tense on palpation
- Pain out of proportion to the clinical picture despite appropriate analgesia is by far the most important sign. Pain is typically deep, severe, and poorly localised. Pain is exacerbated on passive stretch of the compartment
- Paraesthesia, pulseless leg, pallor, 'perishingly cold', paralysis – all late signs and associated with ischaemia and thus poor outcome. Compartment syndrome should be picked up before these signs manifest.

AAPS

- Urgent high-strength analgesia and immediate escalation to the registrar on call are vital in this case and should be stressed in your assessment.

History, Notes, Investigation
- Clear documentation of time pain of onset.
- Review drug chart and analgesia requirement – regional anaesthesia may have masked earlier symptoms.
- Consider using Doppler to help identify pulses.

Preliminary and Further Management
- Keep the patient NBM. Prep for theatre (see Section 9.2).
- As per the BOA standards, this patient needs all circumferential dressings relieved and the limb to be elevated to the level of the heart. The patient should be re-evaluated within 30 minutes and if symptoms persist then they should proceed to urgent operative management within one hour. This patient requires a two-incision, four-compartment fasciotomy. After resolution of compartment syndrome, plastic surgery input may be required to achieve soft tissue coverage [1].

What is the sequence of events leading to compartment syndrome?
Critical elevation of pressure within a closed osteofascial compartment compresses the structures within this compartment. Compression of venous outflow further increases pressure in the compartment and leads to a vicious cycle. Traversing nerves are compressed next, causing the sensory deficit. Tissue necrosis, nerve injury, and muscular infarct occur within 6–10 hours due to lack of microvascular inflow to compressed tissues. Treatment is urgent decompression of the compartment.

How is an abnormal compartment pressure calculated?
In theory a manometer may be used to monitor compartment pressures by measuring the resistance present when saline solution is injected into the compartment. If pressure in the lower limb is >30 mmHg or the pressure is within 30 mmHg of the diastolic pressure, then compartment syndrome can be diagnosed. Normal lower limb compartment pressure is <8 mmHg. In reality, compartment syndrome is a clinical diagnosis and compartment pressures are not usually measured in awake patients – there is a role for this in intubated patients where there is a suspicion of compartment syndrome and the patient cannot communicate their pain.

What are the possible causes of compartment syndrome?
Traumatic causes (fracture, crush injury, thermal injury with circumferential burns), iatrogenic causes (tight circumferential casting and dressing), reperfusion injury, and intracompartmental haemorrhage are all possible causes.

What are the four compartments of the lower leg? What structures are located within each compartment?
- Anterior compartment (anterior tibial artery/vein, deep peroneal nerve, EHL, EDL, tibialis anterior, peroneus tertius)
- Lateral compartment (superficial peroneal nerve, peroneus longus, and brevis)
- Superficial posterior compartment (sural nerve, gastroc, soleus, plantaris)
- Deep posterior compartment (posterior tibial artery/vein, tibial nerve, FHL, FDL, tibialis posterior, popliteus)

Reference

1. BOA (n.d.). 'BOAST – Diagnosis and management of compartment syndrome of the limbs'. Website, www.boa.ac.uk, www.boa.ac.uk/resource/boast-10-pdf.htm.

9.22 Epistaxis

You are the ENT CT1 on call and are called to the emergency department to review a 67-year-old male patient presenting with brisk unilateral epistaxis. The patient is alert, distressed, but otherwise looks well. Observations in the Emergency Department are HR 95, BP 120/80, Sats 98% on room air, RR 16 and temperature 36.6°C. They have a background of hypertension and take aspirin and a statin for peripheral arterial disease. How do you proceed?

Before you begin: Epistaxis varies in severity from self-limiting nosebleeds to life-threatening haemorrhage. Patients need urgent review as the volume of epistaxis is frequently underestimated particularly as bleeding posteriorly can be easily ingested. It is important to triage if there is a traumatic aetiology involved requiring a full ATLS assessment – epistaxis may serve as a distractor from significant intra-cranial or craniomaxillofacial injuries.

A–E

Airway

- Sit the patient up, lean them forward, and ask them to spit blood out. This helps quantify bleeding rate and prevents the patient swallowing blood, which causes nausea.
- Any concerns about airway patency should be escalated to anaesthetics immediately. It is useful to have Yankauer suction to hand to remove large clots in the oropharynx.

Breathing
Circulation

- Haemodynamic stability is a marker of bleeding severity, and if the patient is shocked then start resuscitation and get help early. Note this man has hypertension so the apparent normotension may represent a significant drop in BP for them – starting resuscitation may be appropriate.
- Obtain wide bore IV access in each ACF and take a full set of bloods to include a VBG, FBC, clotting screen and group and save.
- Begin epistaxis haemorrhage management (see below).
- Consider IV tranexamic acid*.

*A Cochrane review in 2018 advised that tranexamic acid may help to stop bleeding at the time of initial administration, preventing the need for more invasive treatments such as cautery and nasal packing [1]

Disability
Exposure
- Perform a full clinical examination, looking for signs of coagulopathy or other underlying diseases. This should include a thorough examination of the nose with headlight and Thudicum speculum, as well as examination of the oropharynx.

AAPS
- Epistaxis not settling with packing, causing haemodynamic compromise, or airway concerns, should all be discussed urgently with the ENT registrar on call.

History, Notes, Investigations
- A focused clinical history including history of epistaxis, possible triggers (e.g. nose-picking, recent nasal procedure, rhinitis, known granulomatous disease), previous bleeding concerns (prior major haemorrhage, bruising, family history of coagulopathy), and any anticoagulant medication.
- Check their notes to see if they have had previous bleeding issues, and if there are baseline bloods on the system.

Preliminary Management
1. First aid: firmly pinch the lower third of the nose, for at least 10 minutes, sit the patient up and lean them forward, telling them to spit out blood. If available, apply ice to the top of nose, or ask the patient to suck on an ice cube.
2. If this fails to improve bleeding, suction nose to remove clots and apply local anaesthetic/decongestant spray or soaked cotton balls to the nose and pinch again for 10 minutes ('blue spray' refers to co-phenylcaine, a mixture of lidocaine with phenylephrine, which serves a similar function and is commonly used in these situations). This will help vasoconstrict the bleeding vessel. After this, examine the nose with a nasal speculum and head torch and consider silver nitrate cautery if a bleeding point is visible – do not cauterise both sides of septum as there is risk of perforation.
3. If bleeding is brisk and ongoing, consider packing the nose with a nasal tampon, for example a Rapid Rhino. Consider antibiotics as per local protocols. A contralateral pack can be considered if a unilateral pack is unsuccessful.
4. If bleeding persists, posterior packing may be needed. This involves inserting a longer tampon, or use of a balloon catheter. At this point it would certainly be prudent to have escalated to the on-call ENT registrar even if the patient is stable, particularly if you have not inserted one of these before.

Further Management
- In bleeding refractory to the above, surgical or interventional management is required - for example sphenopalatine artery ligation.
- Patients who have nasal packs inserted will need admission.
- Consider if the patient's aspirin should be stopped temporarily – note there is usually no benefit to doing this if the bleeding has stopped with anterior packing, although

this should be managed on a case-by-case basis with discussion with haematology as required.
– Consider a 10-day course of topical Naseptin TDS.
– Depending on risk factors such as the patient's age and previous epistaxis history, it would be wise to perform flexible nasendoscopy after the acute event to rule out bleeding secondary to a mass in the nose or nasopharynx.

What is the aetiology of epistaxis?
Seventy-five per cent of cases are idiopathic. Split the remaining causes into local causes such as trauma, irritation, vascular malformation, or malignancy, and systemic causes such as impaired coagulation due to medications, clotting factor deficiencies, and HTN.

What is the blood supply to the nasal septum and how is this relevant in epistaxis?
Blood supply to nasal septum consists of the following arteries: greater palatine (maxillary), anterior ethmoidal (ophthalmic), sphenopalatine (maxillary), posterior ethmoidal (ophthalmic), and septal branch of superior labial (facial) – [mnemonic for these: 'GASPS']. Posterior bleeds typically affect older patients and arise from branches of the sphenopalatine, which is the most common vessel to require ligation.

Which patients require admission?
All patients who need nasal packing should be admitted because they run the risk of hypoxia, inhalation of blood, and ongoing bleeding. If epistaxis resolves with cautery, monitor for at least an hour prior to discharge.

What self-care advice can be given?
Avoid hot drinks, blowing or picking your nose, and alcohol for at least 24 hours. Ensure patients are aware of the first aid measures to implement if this happens again, and that if these do not control the bleeding they should return to hospital.

How do you reverse anticoagulants in an emergency?
Reversal depends on what medication is used, and how severe the bleeding is. Consult hospital guidelines and get haematology input where appropriate. When warfarin requires reversal, this should be guided by severity of the bleeding and what the INR is. In the most severe cases, stop warfarin, administer IV vitamin K, and consider the use of prothrombin complex concentrate or fresh frozen plasma. Other reversal agents are listed below (Table 9.4)

Table 9.4 Reversal agents for commonly used anticoagulants

Medication	Reversal agent
Dabigatran	Praxbind (idarucizumab)
Heparin	Protamine
Rivaroxaban/apixaban	Andexxa (Andexanet alfa) – if available*

* NICE guidelines (2021) state that this is only recommended as an option in those with life-threatening uncontrolled bleeding from the GI tract [2].

References

1. Joseph J, Martinez-Devesa P, Bellorini J, Burton MJ (31 December 2018). 'Tranexamic acid for patients with nasal haemorrhage (epistaxis)'. *Cochrane Database of Systematic Reviews*. Website, www.cochrane.org/CD004328/ENT_tranexamic-acid-help-treat-nosebleeds-epistaxis.

2. NICE (n.d.). 'Andexanet alfa for reversing anticoagulation from apixaban or rivaroxaban | Guidance | NICE'. Website, www.nice.org.uk, www.nice.org.uk/guidance/ta697/chapter/1-Recommendations.

9.23 Thermal Trauma

You are the on-call plastic surgery SHO in a regional burns unit and are called to resus to assess a 37-year-old woman who has been blue-lighted to hospital after being extracted from a housefire. They have a large burn involving the left side of their chest, left arm, and left thigh. Please describe how you would assess this patient.

Before you begin: Thermal trauma should be managed in an ATLS fashion to ensure concomitant injuries are not missed. In reality, it would be unlikely that there would be time to also talk through a major ATLS pathology as well as a major burn. Management of the burn itself should follow EMSB (Emergency Management of Severe Burns) principles. Perform your C–A–E assessment while simultaneously stopping the burn. This is a tough station – but one you could really stand out in, if you are well prepared.

Stopping the Burn

- Completely remove any clothing not stuck to the patient – don't peel off adherent clothing – and brush off any dry chemicals.
- Decontaminate the burn area with copious fluid irrigation. Ideally this should be at 15°C for 20 minutes, then cover to prevent hypothermia. First aid measures are effective within three hours following the burn injury.

A–E
C-Spine
Airway

- Assess for inhalational injury which can cause laryngeal oedema. Concerning features include singed eyebrows/nasal hair, soot around nostrils, swelling of lips, stridor.
- In severe burns or those involving the face, anaesthetics must be involved urgently for consideration of early intubation.

Breathing

- Expose the chest and examine for adequate chest expansion. Look for circumferential burns which can impair inspiration – these may need urgent escharotomy.
- Provide supplemental O_2, 15 L through a non-rebreather mask.
- If there are concerns about carbon monoxide exposure, then perform ABG; remember that O_2 sats are unreliable following carbon monoxide exposure and the true partial pressure of O_2 from an ABG is required.

Circulation

- Insert two large bore intravenous cannulae through unburnt skin. Take off a full set of bloods including a U&Es for a renal baseline, as well as FBC, clotting, carboxyhaemoglobin level, and group and saves.
- Fluid resuscitation to replace ongoing losses from capillary leak due to inflammation. Fluid resuscitation based on the BSA should be started for all burns >20% BSA (>10% in children). BSA calculation and burn depth assessment are discussed below.
- Excess fluid requirements are calculated using the Parkland formula. Hartmann's can be used for fluid requirements. Note that in children, maintenance fluids will also be needed on top of this requirement and are typically given as 5% glucose with 0.45% saline.

> **Modified Parkland formula (as per British Burns Association):**
> 3 × Weight (kg) × Burn surface area (%) = volume replacement in first 24 hours in mls
> (50% given in the first 8 hours, 50% given in the next 16 hours)

- Strict urine output monitoring via a catheter is essential; adults should be aiming for 0.5 ml/kg/hour and paediatric patients <30 kg for 1.0 ml/kg/hour.
- ECG as hypoxia or electrolyte derangement can give dysrhythmias.
- Check circulation in each limb to ensure that there are no circumferential burns that require escharotomy. Doppler can be used to assess pulses if needed.

Disability

- Regular GCS reassessment – carbon monoxide can give a delayed fall in conscious level.
- Control the patient's temperature through active and passive means.

Exposure

- Fully expose the patient by removing all jewellery and clothing to assess the total body surface area and depth of the burn whilst keeping the patient warm. Methods of calculating TBSA and burn depth are described below.
- Top-to-toe examination, including log roll if required.

AAPS

- Given the area affected, strong analgesia such as IV morphine will likely be required. Senior support is essential in this case.
- Given her age a pregnancy test must also be performed.

History, Notes, Investigations

- A burns history using an AMPLE framework, including identifying duration and nature of thermal exposure, clothing that was worn, and what local first aid was provided.
- Imaging of any concomitant injuries that have been identified.

Preliminary Management
- Clinical photography with the patient's consent.
- Tetanus (N.B. routine use of prophylactic antibiotics is not recommended).
- Dressing with non-adhesive layers and absorbent dressings.
- Ongoing fluid resuscitation and patient warming (e.g. with a Bair hugger) as above.
- NG tubes are typically inserted for larger burns.
- Escharotomy if required.

Further Management
- Transfer of patient to appropriate burns unit (if required).
- MDT approach to manage the local and systemic complications of burns.
- Surgical approaches in the acute phase involve early tangential excision and grafting of burns.
- For larger burns, skin substitutes can be applied to the wound bed until autologous skin becomes available.

How is BSA calculated?
Wallace's rule of 9s or the palmar 1% rule can be used as a rough guide. For more accurate estimates, a Lund and Browder chart can be used.

How is burn depth assessed?
Burns are assessed clinically noting the colour, capillary refill, sensation, and presence of blisters. Superficial burns are blanching, non-blistered, painful areas of erythema. Superficial partial thickness burns are painful, with a pink 'moist' appearance with blistering. Deep partial thickness burns have fixed (non-blanching) 'cherry red' staining, with reduced sensation and no blistering. Full thickness burns have a white or 'leathery' appearance, no blisters or blanching, and are insensate. Many burns will have areas of differing depths, and the depths can evolve over time.

When should burns be transferred to a regional burns centre?
The National Network for Burn Care in the UK have produced nationally agreed guidelines, endorsed by the British Burn Association, regarding which patients should have early consultation with a burn service [1]. These include (but are not limited to):
- TBSA >3% in adults (>2% in children)
- Burns involving face, hands, feet, genitalia, perineum, and large joints
- Full thickness burns
- Burns of chemical or electrical nature
- Circumferential burns
- Burns in the elderly, very young, or those with medical comorbidities

What complications should you be aware of when managing thermal trauma?
Complications can be split into local and systemic. Local complications include scarring and contractures which in turn cause poor cosmesis, stiffening of the tissues, and a decreased range of motion. Systemic complications can include rhabdomyolysis, acute respiratory distress syndrome, Curling's ulcers, AKI caused by hypotension, and myoglobinuria.

What form of grafting could be used to cover the damaged skin?
Given a relatively large area is involved, a split thickness skin graft would most likely be used. These can be meshed to allow an even larger area to be covered.

What are the advantages and disadvantages of a full thickness skin graft?
Full thickness skin grafts are harvested with the entire epidermis and dermis. These grafts can give a better cosmetic outcome, and contract less than STSGs. However, thicker grafts require better blood supplies at the recipient sites, and the donor site will require primary closure.

Reference

1. National Network for Burn Care (NNBC) (February 2012). 'National Burn Care Referral Guidance Specialised Services National Network for Burn Care (NNBC) National Burn Care Referral Guidance 2'. Website, www.britishburnassociation.org/wp-content/uploads/2018/02/National-Burn-Care-Referral-Guidance-2012.pdf.

9.24 Right Iliac Fossa Pain

You are the on-call general surgical CT2. You are called to the emergency department to assess a 19-year-old girl complaining of severe right iliac fossa pain for the last two hours. She is nauseous with HR 110, BP 110/75, RR 16, Sats 99% on RA, temperature 37.9°C. How do you proceed?

Before you begin: Ensure you have a clear differential for acute abdominal pain. A full differential list is covered in Section 9.7. However, this should be tailored to specific scenarios based on the patient's sex, age, and location of pain. For this scenario:

- GI causes: appendicitis, Meckel's diverticulitis, IBD, hernia-related pathology, bowel ischaemia, obstruction, perforation, constipation.
- Renal causes: ureteric colic, pyelonephritis.
- Gynaecological causes: ovarian torsion/rupture, ectopic pregnancy, Mittelschmerz, endometriosis, pelvic inflammatory disease.

Remember, all scenarios in which there are concerns about infection should have SEPSIS 6 initiated – labour this point to the examiners.

A–E
Airway
Breathing
- High-flow oxygen to keep patient in the range 94%–98%.

Circulation
- Remember that young people are better able to compensate physiologically so do not be fooled by a relatively normal blood pressure, the patient may still be very unwell, so ensure you have wide bore IV access in each ACF and begin fluid resuscitation and consider catheterisation.
- Take a full set of bloods including FBC, U&Es, LFTs, clotting and group and saves with a mind to potential operative management. Blood cultures and VBG are needed as part of SEPSIS 6.

Disability
Exposure
- Full abdominal examination including hernial orifices and PR.
- Pelvic exam if appropriate given earlier findings in a male a testicular examination would be required.)

AAPS
- Pregnancy test is particularly important in this situation – if positive this may represent an ectopic pregnancy, necessitating urgent gynaecological input.

History, Notes, Investigation
- AMPLE history should be taken, before eliciting features indicative of appendicitis, such as nausea, vomiting (although vomiting more than once or twice is rare), and migratory pain to McBurney's point. Other relevant factors include age, and risk factors such as poor fibre intake and smoking.
- Full gynae and sexual history given the patient's age.
- Urine dip (in appendicitis expect LEU positive and NIT negative).
- Based on clinical findings, USS or CT can be used to reduce the rate of negative appendectomy. USS is the preferred imaging strategy in this scenario (given they are a young female), with CT or diagnostic laparoscopy performed if the appendix cannot be visualised on US. Note that appendicitis remains a clinical diagnosis, and imaging is not required to take the patient to theatre.
- If there are concerns regarding gynaecological pathology, then gynae review ± transvaginal ultrasound is sensible.

The history and examination reveal appendicitis as the presumptive diagnosis. What are the clinical signs of appendicitis?
Clinical signs of appendicitis include:
- Rovsing's sign (palpating LIF causes reproduction of pain in the RIF due to peritoneal irritation).
- Rebound tenderness.
- Percussion pain over McBurney's point (one-third of the distance from the ASIS to umbilicus).
- Guarding.
- Psoas sign (RIF pain elicited by extension or flexion of right hip against resistance).
- Obturator sign (RIF pain from internal or external rotation of the rotated hip).

The clinical examination is suspicious for appendicitis. How is appendicitis managed?
- Resuscitate, ensure full SEPSIS 6 management complete (commence antibiotics as per local protocol), begin operative workup (see Section 9.2).
- Laparoscopic appendicectomy is the gold standard for management of uncomplicated appendicitis. There is a poorly defined role for the use of

nonoperative management – primarily, antibiotics. This is a decision for the admitting senior surgeon.
- If the appendix has perforated, it may be managed nonoperatively with antibiotics ± interval appendectomy.
- If the appendicitis has formed an appendix mass/peri-appendicular abscess, then this can be treated surgically, or conservatively with intravenous antibiotics and possible percutaneous drainage.

What is the pathological sequence of events typically leading to acute appendicitis
The appendiceal lumen becomes obstructed (e.g. by faecolith or lymphoid tissue hyperplasia), resulting in bacterial overgrowth, inflammation of the appendix, reduced venous drainage, and subsequent ischaemia. Perforation can occur as the appendicular artery (branch of the ileocecal artery) can become thrombosed, resulting in gangrene and perforation.

In what position does the inflamed appendix usually lie?
Most commonly retrocaecal (74%) followed by pelvic (21%). It can also lie in the pre and post ileal, paracaecal, and subcaecal positions.

Can patients be managed nonoperatively?
While laparoscopic appendicectomy is the gold standard treatment for uncomplicated appendicitis, it has been noted that in patients without complicating clinical or radiological features, nonoperative management antibiotics and fluids can be a safe and effective approach although there is a recurrence risk of almost 40% after five years [1].

What scoring systems can be used to diagnose appendicitis?
Appendicitis is a clinical diagnosis but there are several scoring systems, including the Alvarado score, the Appendicitis Inflammatory Response (AIR) score, and the Adult Appendicitis Score (AAS), which can serve as adjuncts. These calculate a score based on a mixture of clinical and laboratory features. These scores can help to exclude acute appendicitis, accurately identifying low-risk patients, and decrease the negative appendectomy rates in such patients.

Reference

1. Di Saverio S, Podda M, De Simone B, Ceresoli M, Augustin G, Gori A, et al. (2020). 'Diagnosis and treatment of acute appendicitis: 2020 update of the WSES Jerusalem guidelines'. *World Journal of Emergency Surgery* 15(1): 27, https://doi.org/10.1186/s13017-020-00306-3.

9.25 Paediatric Trauma

You are the orthopaedic CT1 and are called to the emergency department to assess a seven-year-old boy who has been thrown sideways off his bike after colliding with a rock. He fell on his outstretched right hand with his arm extended, and experienced sudden onset severe pain. He is now holding his right elbow, which is swollen. He has been crying from the pain. His observations are stable. How do you proceed?

Before you begin: The most likely diagnosis here is a supracondylar fracture– ensure a paediatric trauma call is placed as a full assessment to identify concomitant injuries is required. Ensure your senior is made aware. Remark on your awareness that there are different physiological parameters and different medications/dosages used in paediatric trauma, and that you would rely on support from your paediatric colleagues where required. *General points about paediatric trauma which may be relevant to these scenarios are highlighted in italics.* Highlighting your communication with the patient and reassurance of the parent/carer should feature in the A–E. Always mention you would consider non-accidental injury.

A–E
C-Spine
Airway
– *A crying child likely has a patent airway.*

Breathing
Circulation
– *Ask for a full set of observations, bearing in mind the normal range varies by age and that children have a high physiological reserve that can mask blood loss.*
– *For fluids/meds you would use weight-based dosing.*
– *In a smaller child, where necessary, you could use a resuscitation tape to estimate weight from length.*

Disability
Exposure
– Full top-to-toe examination with look, feel, move approach to examination of the upper limb. Document a clear neurovascular assessment of the anterior interosseous nerve, median, radial, and ulnar nerves.
– Check the hand for features of vascular compromise (pallor, prolonged CRT, reduced or absent pulses, cool temperature).
– Differentials also include distal humerus or olecranon fracture, subluxation of the radial head. Plain radiographs will help here.
– *Hypothermia can rapidly develop in children, so ensure they are adequately warmed if you are exposing the patient.*

AAPS
– Ensure adequate analgesia – paracetamol, ibuprofen, Entonox and intranasal diamorphine are often used in the paediatric cases.

History, Notes, Investigation
– AMPLE history. Always remember the possibility of non-accidental injury – try to get a history from child where possible (even if further history is obtained from the parent) and consider child safeguarding review if needed.
– Plain film radiograph (AP and lateral) to check for fracture. Other signs to look for with supracondylar fractures include the posterior fat pad (sign of haemarthrosis and

possible occult fracture), and displacement of the anterior humeral line (should intersect middle third of capitellum). Imaging will help determine Gartland classification.

- CT imaging can be sought to further characterise fracture and aid preoperative planning (rarely used in practice).

Preliminary and Further Management

- Fractures are classified by the Gartland classification (type 1–4) based the nature of injury and the level of displacement.
- Gartland type 1 fractures are usually managed nonoperatively with long arm casting with the elbow in less than 90 degrees of flexion for three to four weeks with repeat XR at one week to check for displacement.
- Gartland type 2 + are usually immobilised by splinting in a position of comfort (with a neurovascular assessment before and after this) and then listed for theatre for operative fixation.

How would you assess the distal neurological function in a child?
In a child, the motor examinations of the relevant nerves can be conveniently grouped into 'rock, paper, scissors, OK.' Making a fist (rock) tests the median nerve, straightening the fingers (paper) tests the radial nerve, lateral abduction of the fingers (scissors) tests the ulnar nerve, and making the OK sign tests the anterior interosseus nerve (a branch of the median nerve supplying the deep flexors which must always be assessed in supracondylar fracture). Sensation of the dorsal aspect first webspace (radial nerve), tip of index finger (median nerve), and tip of little finger (ulnar nerve) should also be checked.

For those requiring operative management, how long can you wait before operating?
As per BOA standards, surgery should be carried out on the day of the injury. Those with no deficit do not need to go to theatre overnight; however, patients with concerns about vascular compromise, threatened skin viability, or open injuries require urgent surgery [1].

The child proceeds to closed reduction and percutaneous pinning. What complications should the parents be aware of during consenting?
Generic complications include bleeding, infection, pain, stiffness, malunion/non-union, need for metalwork removal, and compartment syndrome. Specific complications would include a risk of nerve palsies, particularly the anterior interosseous nerve injury from the fracture itself and ulnar nerve injury if medially placed K-wires are used. A feared complication is Volkmann's ischaemic contracture, which produces a permanent flexion deformity of the wrist and a claw-like hand.

What are some signs in the history or exam that would make you suspicious of non-accidental injury in a child?
History: repeated or delayed presentations to the emergency department with trauma injuries, discordance between history and severity or nature of injury, history inconsistent between adult and child, parents not complying with medical advice or behaving strangely in ED, implausible mechanism of injury given patient's age (rolling age around four months, pulling to stand around nine months).

Examination: bruises in different stages of healing, previous evidence of multiple injuries or fractures, bruising of/behind ears or other unusual locations (e.g. inner thighs, torso), torn frenulum – always look in the mouth, injury to genitalia or perineum, retinal haemorrhage, as well as common abuse injuries such as bites, and cigarette or iron burns.

Reference

1. BOA (n.d.). 'BOAST – Supracondylar fractures in the humerus in children'. Website, www.boa.ac.uk, accessed 19 Feb. 2024, www.boa.ac.uk/resource/boast-11-pdf.html.

9.26 Back Pain

You are the orthopaedic SHO on call and have been called to the emergency department to review a 71-year-old male patient who has noted he is unable to pass urine. He reports acute lower back pain. He has no significant past medical history of note and is haemodynamically stable. How would you proceed?

Before you begin: The vignette should make you concerned for cauda equina syndrome (CES). This is a surgical emergency which can rapidly progress to profoundly debilitating complications – prompt diagnosis and management is essential. The history of urinary retention and back pain could also represent prostate cancer which in turn can metastasise to the spine.

A–E

You have already been told the patient is haemodynamically stable. Therefore, you should confirm the patient has no life-threatening pathology with an A–E approach before moving on to more fully assess the patient.

Exposure

- A comprehensive examination of lower limb neurology, including a straight leg raise, and gait assessment, should be performed to help identify features of cauda equina (see below). The use of an ASIA neurological assessment form is recommended.
- PR examination should be performed to assess for anal tone, deep rectal sensation, perianal light touch, and to also check for a malignant feeling prostate (hard, lumpy, asymmetrical).
- Spinal examination including assessing for midline point tenderness.

AAPS

- Escalate to your senior to make them aware of the situation. Concerns about CES should be referred for urgent neurosurgical input.

History, Notes, Investigation

- History to elicit if there has been a change in bladder/bowel function, or lack of sensation on passing urine/faeces or on wiping oneself after going to the toilet, incontinence, new sexual dysfunction, change in motor and sensation, and bilateral leg pain.

- History of prostate symptoms (prostate cancer), fevers (spinal abscess), weight loss (other cancers). History of CES symptoms.
- A pre- and post-void bladder scan is essential to help demonstrate urinary retention. Note that classically CES presents with painless retention (the bladder is insensate).
- Lumbar sacral MRI without contrast for suspected CES – if not available then urgently discuss with radiology and local neurosurgical services regarding your available options including transfer to a centre with ability to perform MRI.

Classical signs and symptoms of cauda equina syndrome

- Bilateral sciatica
- Bilateral sensory or motor abnormalities which are severe or progressive, gait disturbances
- Saddle sensory changes
- Urinary: retention, reduced power of voiding, impaired sensation of urinary flow, incontinence
- Bowel: impaired sensation of rectal fullness, laxity of anal sphincter, incontinence
- Sexual dysfunction

Preliminary Management
- Catheterise patients who are in retention and record the urine volume drained. Whether the patient can feel a 'catheter tug' is another useful assessment.

Further Management
- Definitive management requires decompression of the cause of CES, such as laminectomy, discectomy, abscess drainage, or tumour debulking.

What is the most likely cause of CES in this situation?
Disc herniation represents the most common cause of CES, although given the patient is a male in his 70s, you should be concerned also about prostate cancer with metastatic spread to the spine. Other causes include trauma, infection (such as discitis, epidural abscess, or Pott's disease), and other cancers.

Which cancers typically metastasise to the spine?
Thyroid, prostate, renal, lung, and breast (remembered as 'These Pathologies Really Love Bone', also as paired structure/organs either side of the midline). In the case of prostate cancer, it is due to the venous drainage of the prostate which connects with the vertebral venous plexus.

9.27 Trauma in Pregnancy
You are the general surgical CT2 on call at a DGH overnight and are called to assess a 24-year-old female who is 32 weeks pregnant. She has fallen off a ladder at home and has been brought in by ambulance. She complains of constant abdominal pain, has not felt her baby moving since the accident, and has noticed extended bruising across her upper abdomen. Her observations are HR 105, BP 102/68, RR 14, Sats 95% on RA, apyrexial. How do you proceed?

Before you begin: It would be scary to be confronted with a trauma in pregnancy case in an interview – you may have minimal trauma experience, and even less in obstetric trauma. Based on previous experience, this is an unlikely scenario, but is a good way to assess the principles you have learned in this book thus far. You aren't expected to be an obstetric trauma expert, so take things back to basic principles and remember your role is to complete a thorough A–E and show you are safe. You have two patients to manage in this trauma scenario; however, the principle during initial management remains to resuscitate the mother. The physiology of the mother is altered during pregnancy, and the foetus has its own physiology. You will need obstetric help and should ask for them to be contacted as early as possible (they would typically be present from the start for a trauma call of this nature). This case will require very clear communication with the mother, so assigning a member of the team to stay at the top of the bed with her may be prudent. We would suggest candidates read the relevant chapter in the ATLS manual to prepare. Our assessment below will highlight some *key general points in italics* to be aware of in a maternal trauma setting.

A–E
C-Spine
Airway
Breathing
–   *Note that ABGs in pregnancy would normally show hypocapnia (due to greater maternal tidal volume) – a normal CO_2 may therefore be concerning. Consider high-flow oxygen early to counteract rapid deoxygenation.*

Circulation
–   IV access, full set of bloods including clotting and Rhesus status of the mother, IV fluid resuscitation, and activation of the obstetric major haemorrhage protocol if there is suspicion of internal haemorrhage which is greater than 500 mls and not controlled.
–   The uterus should be displaced to the left to decompress the vena cava – this can be done by logrolling the patient to 15–30 degrees to their left side and supporting the right side.
–   FAST scan including a basic transabdominal ultrasound (looking for foetal heart, position and lie of the baby, as well as assessing for foetal movements) are both useful investigations, as is continuous foetal monitoring with CTG (this will be performed by the obstetric team). Note at this stage a differential of placental abruption, uterine rupture or acute hypovolaemia causing foetal bradycardia (via placental hypoperfusion) should be considered.
–   *Blood volume increases in pregnancy and therefore higher blood volumes can be lost before signs of hypovolaemia are exhibited – foetal distress may develop before these signs do. Early and vigorous resuscitation is therefore key.*

Disability
–   Don't mistake pre-eclampsia for head injury; obtain urine dip.

Exposure

- Full top-to-toe examination including a log roll to identify concomitant pathology. Carefully examine the abdomen looking for signs of abruption, uterine rupture, and peritoneal irritation manifesting in the form of peritonitis (combined with basic obstetric TA scan).
- PV examination should be performed – ideally by obstetric team. Delivery may be indicated in cases of uterine rupture or placental abruption. It is also essential to deliver if this would improve the chances of maternal survival as this relieves the cardiac afterload significantly.

AAPS

History, Notes, Investigations

- AMPLE history including circumstances of the fall. Be vigilant for any concerns about domestic violence (see below).
- Imaging of any further injuries identified and investigations regarding cause of the fall.

Preliminary Management

- Ongoing fluid resuscitation.
- Rhesus Ig as required (if mother is Rh-negative).
- If risk of pre-term labour, call neonatology.
- Alert obstetric HDU if patient needs higher-level care.

Further Management

- Decisions about emergency C-section should be made by the obstetric team. The analgesia of choice should be GA and not spinal due to probable haemodynamic instability. Early escalation to neonatology is required here as you anticipate a compromised foetus.

What are the primary causes of foetal mortality in trauma?
The most common cause is maternal shock/death, hence the importance of maternal resuscitation. Other causes include placenta abruption and uterine rupture.

What signs may point you towards placental abruption?
PV bleeding, a tender woody uterus, frequent uterine contractions or tetany, and uterine irritability when palpated are all signs of placental abruption.

How should a Rhesus-negative mother be managed in this scenario?
All Rhesus-negative mothers presenting with trauma anywhere near the uterus should receive Rh immunoglobulins within 72 hours.

In addition to your own seniors, who else would you like to have assess the patient or be aware of the patient to help manage this case?

- Trauma team
- Obstetrics team ± obstetric HDU/ITU

- Neonatology
- For operative management: theatre coordinator, obstetric anaesthetist.

What normal physiological changes occur during pregnancy that may be relevant in an acute scenario like this?

- Maternal heart rate rises and blood pressure falls during pregnancy (returning to near normal levels by term).
- Circulating blood volume increases up to about 34 weeks – mothers can lose 1–1.5 L of blood before hypovolaemic signs are exhibited, but foetal distress may present before this.
- Increasing tidal volume decreases CO_2 levels, so hypocapnia is common until late pregnancy.
- Pregnant women can become hypoxic more readily due to altered lung function, diaphragmatic splinting, and increased oxygen consumption, therefore high flow supplemental oxygen should be administered early where necessary to counteract rapid deoxygenation.

What features may make you concerned about inter-partner violence?

- Incongruent history and examination.
- Isolated injuries to gravid abdomen or multiple bruises in the abdomen and back not justified by the mechanism of trauma.
- Multiple presentations to ED/doctor.
- Diminished self-worth/mental health concerns/substance use.
- Partner insisting on presence during consultations.

9.28 Epigastric Pain

You are the on-call surgical CT1 called to the emergency department to review a 51-year-old woman who has presented with constant epigastric pain and persistent vomiting. She has previously suffered from intermittent bouts of colicky right-sided upper abdominal pain but has never had anything like this before. Observations are HR 115, BP 105/75, RR 16, Sats 91% on room air, afebrile. How do you proceed?

Before you begin: As discussed before, a well-rehearsed abdominal pain differential is something you should have at your disposal. Given this pathology is epigastric, weight your differential more heavily in favour of upper GI causes, while including medical causes such as MI and lower lobe pneumonia. The preceding history should be concerning for biliary colic – this pain may therefore represent acute cholecystitis, cholangitis, or pancreatitis (likely secondary to a biliary stone).

A–E

Airway
Breathing
- Assess for signs of respiratory pathology. Start high-flow oxygen.

Circulation

- Tachycardia and hypotension necessitate wide bore IV access in each ACF, full bloods workup including lipase/amylase and LFTs to help determine cause, as well as calcium, urea, LDH, albumin, and ABG to allow pancreatitis severity scoring (Glasgow score), and fluid resuscitation.
- Catheterise to facilitate strict fluid balance monitoring.

Disability

- Significant fever may point to cholangitis.
- CBG measurement is required for Glasgow score of pancreatitis severity.

Exposure

- Full abdominal examination looking for signs of pancreatitis (epigastric tenderness, evidence of third spacing such as basal lung crepitations, evidence of retroperitoneal bleed such as Grey Turner and Cullen's signs, Chvostek's sign), acute cholecystitis (Murphy's sign), and cholangitis (jaundice).

AAPS

- Antiemetics would be prudent.

History, Notes, Investigation

- Pancreatitis: pain history – pancreatitis pain classically radiates to the back and is relieved by sitting forwards. Identify possible causes and risk factors, for example alcohol intake, previous gallstones, trauma or recent ERCP. N.B. in the interview, it is better to list the top three to four most likely causes rather than list the full 'I GET SMASHED' mnemonic (idiopathic, gallstones, ethanol, trauma, steroids, mumps, autoimmune, scorpion stings, hypercalcaemia/hypertriglyceridaemia, ERCP, drugs/medications – such as azathioprine, thiazides).
- Erect CXR to exclude pneumoperitoneum secondary to perforated viscous.
- USS biliary system to identify stones, duct dilation, and radiological signs of acute cholecystitis. Note that a CT scan is typically not used in pancreatitis until 48–72 hours after symptom onset (as radiological evidence of complications is more likely to be present at this point), although a CT with IV contrast would be used if there are concerns about GI perforation.

The amylase level comes back as 3,270 IU/L (normal range 40–140 IU/L) and the ultrasound shows a gallstone obstructing the common bile duct. How do you proceed?
These findings confirm my suspicion of pancreatitis secondary to gallstone disease. Pancreatitis patients can be seriously unwell, so I would ensure I provided ample fluid resuscitation and reassessed their A–E, and obtained a senior review, and a critical care outreach team review. I would calculate the patient's PANCREAS score to provide a marker of severity. I would make the patient temporarily NBM and insert an NGT as she is currently vomiting profusely, while being wary that in pancreatitis patients should have oral intake restarted as soon as it is safe to do so. Given this is stone related, an ERCP ±

sphincterotomy may be required, and I would work the patient up for this. Following this, she should be closely monitored for signs of complications of pancreatitis, while having nutritional input as required.

*NICE suggests that enteral nutrition is started within 72 hours for those with severe or moderately severe acute pancreatitis. N.B. NICE guidelines also advise against offering prophylactic antimicrobials to patients with acute pancreatitis [1].

What scoring systems exist for pancreatitis?
The Glasgow-Imrie scoring system [2] is commonly used and is worth learning (the parameters spell PANCREAS) (Table 9.5):

Table 9.5 Glasgow PANCREAS score

PaO2	<59.3 mmHg (7.9 kPa)
Age	>55 years
Neutrophils/WBC	>15 × 10³/μL (10⁹/L)
Calcium	2 mmol/L
Renal (serum urea)	>16 mmol/L
Enzymes (LDH)	>600 IU/L
Albumin	<3.2 g/dL (32 g/L)
Sugar (glucose)	>180 mg/dL (10 mmol/L)

Each category is worth one point, and a score of three or higher indicates high risk for severe pancreatitis requiring high-dependency care. There is also Ranson's criteria for pancreatitis mortality based on initial and 48-hour laboratory values, and the Balthazar scoring system based on radiological appearances.

What complications of pancreatitis are you aware of?
There are local complications, including pancreatic necrosis, pseudocysts, abscesses, portal or splenic vein thromboses, and progression to chronic pancreatitis. There are also systemic complications such as AKI, ARDS, and metabolic disturbances (hyperglycaemia and hypocalcaemia). Pancreatic necrosis will require IV antibiotics ± necrosectomy. Chronic pancreatitis will need nutritional input ± use of CREON supplementation.

How are pancreatic pseudocysts managed?
Pancreatic pseudocysts represent a collection of fluid adjacent to the pancreas (it lacks an epithelial lining, hence the 'pseudo-'). These typically resolve spontaneously, but if they fail to do so, and are symptomatic (e.g. pain, vomiting, or weight loss) then offer endoscopic US-guided drainage, or surgical drainage if this fails.

What signs would make you more worried that this could be ascending cholangitis? How would this be managed?
Ascending cholangitis is typically related to biliary stones. It classically presents with Charcot's triad of upper abdominal pain, fever, and jaundice, and can progress to Reynold's pentad with the addition of confusion and hypotension. These patients can

quickly deteriorate into life-threatening sepsis, so an A–E assessment should be performed, the SEPSIS 6 protocol should be started, and the patient should be prepared for urgent biliary decompression if they continue to deteriorate despite medical management (this is typically with ERCP ± sphincterotomy ± drainage stent).

What signs would point to a perforated peptic ulcer? How would this be managed?
A perforated peptic ulcer would likely have a preceding history (dyspepsia, bloating, reflux) of, and risk factors (*Helicobacter pylori* infection, smoking, alcohol, family history) for, ulcer disease. A perforation typically causes severe diffuse abdominal pain, with tachycardia and abdominal rigidity. The patient should be resuscitated, SEPSIS 6 protocol initiated, and NGT decompression of stomach considered. Erect CXR/lateral decubitus film may show free air. Typically, a CT scan is arranged to confirm diagnosis – if the patient is too unstable for this, they may proceed directly to theatres for surgical repair with omental patching via laparotomy or laparoscopy. Ongoing PPI + risk factor management with *H. pylori* testing ± eradication therapy will be needed after the acute episode.

References

1. NICE. (n.d.). 'Pancreatitis'. Website, www.nice.org.uk/guidance/ng104/chapter/Recommendations#acute-pancreatitis.

2. Blamey SL, Imrie CW, O'Neill J, Gilmour WH, Carter DC (1984). 'Prognostic factors in acute pancreatitis'. *Gut* 25(12): 1340–1346, https://doi.org/10.1136/gut.25.12.1340.

9.29 Leaking Laparotomy Wound

You are the general surgical CT1 covering the ward. You are on your lunch break when the nursing staff bleep you asking you to review a 45-year-old woman who is five days post emergency laparotomy and omental patch repair for a perforated duodenal ulcer. The nurses have noticed fluid soaking through the dressings, and the patient has pain around the wound. How do you proceed?

Before you begin: As with all cases where the nurses are calling you, ask for a set of observations and ensure the patient's notes are available for when you arrive on the ward. Fluid from a wound may simply represent a small amount of 'strikethrough' seen on wounds postoperatively, or it may represent wound infection. However, the most concerning differential is abdominal wound dehiscence. As you cannot rule this out you must urgently review the patient. Prior to interview we would recommend revising the layers of the abdominal wall (both above and below the arcuate line) – in the interest of space, anatomy is left out of this textbook.

A–E
Airway
Breathing
– Beware of the possibility that abdominal pain is splinting the diaphragm. Though worth remarking upon, this would not be life-threatening and would permit you to move on to assessing circulation.

Circulation

- Consider initiating SEPSIS 6 protocol and resuscitation if haemodynamically unstable, as the abdominal wall dehiscence may be driven by an intra-abdominal source (infection, leak, etc.).

Disability

- A temperature may indicate a wound or intra-abdominal infection.

Exposure

- Take down the dressings and examine the wound sites looking for signs of wound dehiscence, including bulging of the wound, increasing wound discharge, and pink serous discharge (representing peritoneal exudate, and a concerning sign of impending complete dehiscence).
- With a sterile gloved finger examine if the rectus sheath is intact or not, to determine if this is superficial or full thickness dehiscence. Removing one or two sutures can help with this.
- Examine for signs of infection of the wound, see if pus can be expressed by gently putting pressure on the sides of the wound.

AAPS

- You should give strong analgesia with an antiemetic to avoid opiate-induced vomiting which would increase intra-abdominal pressure.
- You must get your registrar to review this patient urgently.

History, Notes, Investigations

- Confirm the patient's operation, their postoperative course so far, and the timescale of the fluid leaking.
- Wound swab.

Preliminary Management

- Analgesia and reassurance: seeing an abdominal wound opened is understandably stressful for patients and can be extremely painful.
- Cover in saline-soaked gauze: do not attempt to reduce exposed bowel on the ward.
- Work the patient up for CEPOD (see Section 9.2).
- Commence broad-spectrum antibiotics and fluids.
- Ensure appropriate warming to avoid risk of hypothermia.

Further Management

- In theatres the patient will have debridement of non-viable wound edges and repair with mass closure technique: size 1 sutures are thrown through all layers of the abdominal wall, rectus fascia, and peritoneum, before closing the skin as a separate layer. As per 'Jenkins rule' for abdominal closure, a continuous suture (the length of which should be four times the length of the wound) should be used with 1 cm bites, 1 cm apart.

- If the dehiscence is too large, there is gross peritonitis, or another intra-abdominal procedure is needed, an 'open abdomen' may be left for delayed primary closure later. In these cases, a temporary abdominal closure, for example visceral protection sheet (e.g. Bogotá bag) and negative pressure dressing is used (see below).
- Try to assess and manage causes of dehiscence, such as: malnutrition/ hypoalbuminaemia, infection, hyperglycaemia, increasing intra-abdominal pressure through constipation or coughing.

How would management change if it was superficial dehiscence?
I would ensure my registrar had reviewed the patient to confirm it was not full thickness dehiscence. As the skin has dehisced but the rectus sheath remains intact, the wound can be washed out and then standard wound care measures can be taken to allow the area to heal. Vacuum-assisted dressings are useful in helping large areas heal by secondary intention (although you must be certain there are no areas of full thickness dehiscence or you risk forming an enterocutaneous fistula).

Intraoperatively the wound edges are infected and friable, how does this change management?
The infected wound edges help to explain why the closure has failed. It would be unwise to attempt to suture closed infected tissue – the inflamed and oedematous tissue will be being closed under increased tension, and the friable tissue is less likely to hold the sutures. Moreover, you may be trapping infection under the skin surface. The wound can be left open, classically using a Bogotá bag (a sterile plastic sheet to cover the bowel), while awaiting definitive closure later. Definitive closure may require plastics input for abdominal wall reconstruction, depending on the size of the defect.

What risk factors are there for postoperative wound dehiscence?
I would split these into preoperative, intraoperative, and postoperative factors. Preoperative factors include obesity, diabetes, and poor nutritional state. Intraoperative factors include contamination of the wound site, increased bowel handling (increasing bowel oedema and subsequent intra-abdominal pressure), and poor surgical technique. Postoperative factors would include infection at the surgical site, poor tissue perfusion postoperatively, and causes of raised intra-abdominal pressure such as coughing or constipation.

9.30 Open Fracture
You are the orthopaedic CT1 on call and are called to assess a 19-year-old male who presents with an open wound and visible fractured bone ends after being hit in the shin with a baseball bat during a fight. They are alert and their observations are stable. How would you proceed?

Before you begin: Remember: life before limb. This is an open fracture case, and you should be mentioning BOA open fracture guidelines [1] and the Gustilo–Anderson classification. Open fractures should be managed at a combined orthoplastics centre as per the BOA standards. As with all trauma cases, you should inform your senior on your way to review the patient; ensure a trauma call has been put out.

A–E

C-Spine

- Given the history of a fight, triple immobilise the C-spine with collar, blocks, and tape.

Airway

Breathing

- Given there is trauma due to blunt force, a comprehensive chest assessment as part of your primary survey is important.

Circulation

- Establish IV access. Take bloods with a mind to potential operative management. IV antibiotics should be administered as soon as possible (within one hour).

Disability

Exposure

- Full top-to-toe examination including log roll, then a look, feel, move approach to the affected limb (see Section 9.8). Assess and document neurovascular status; assess dorsalis pedis, posterior tibial arteries, and distal capillary refill time. If not palpable, a Doppler can be used. Any vascular concerns will require an urgent vascular team assessment and a CT angiogram.

AAPS

History, Notes, Investigations

- AMPLE history, determine the nature of any contamination of the wound.
- Orthogonal view XRs of affected area and imaging of other injuries as appropriate (if performing a trauma CT then ensure you request lower limb ± angiography if required).

Preliminary Management

This patient has sustained a high-energy open lower limb fracture and will require an initial debridement within 12 hours as per BOA standards [1] under joint orthoplastics input:

- Keep NBM.
- Remove only visible gross contamination in ED, formal washout should happen in theatre.
- Clinical photography of wound (with patient's consent).
- Cover wound with saline-soaked gauze and occlusive film.
- Reduce the fracture under analgesia or sedation with senior emergency department team support. Splint using an above-knee non-circumferential backslab. Repeat NV assessment after splinting.
- IV abx within one hour.
- Tetanus booster as required.
- Mark and consent.
- Perform and document complete secondary survey.

Further Management

- Combined orthoplastic approach. The patient will need irrigation, debridement, fixation, and soft tissue cover.
- Debride immediately if highly contaminated wounds (e.g. sewage, agricultural, or aquatic contamination) or if there is vascular compromise (compartment syndrome, ischaemia).
- Debride within 12 hours for high-energy solitary open fracture.
- Debride within 24 hours for all other low-energy fractures.
- Internal stabilisation should occur when it can be followed by immediate definitive soft tissue cover. Soft tissue cover should occur within 72 hours if unable to do at the same time as debridement.

How are open fractures classified?

The Gustilo–Anderson classification system is used after initial debridement of open fractures to determine severity, guide management, and predict the likelihood of complications.

An abridged version (suitable for interview) is:

- Type 1: ≤1 cm wound with minimal contamination/muscle damage.
- Type 2: 1–10 cm wound with moderate soft tissue injury.
- Type 3A: >10 cm wound secondary to high-energy trauma, extensive soft tissue damage and contamination, with periosteal stripping.
- Type 3B: as for 3A, but with inadequate soft tissue coverage.
- Type 3C: as for 3B, but with any vascular injury requiring repair.

Note that types 1, 2, and 3A can usually be managed with local soft tissue coverage. Types 3B and 3C often require free or rotational flaps ± vascular repair.

How would management differ if there was a concomitant arterial injury?

During the primary survey, resuscitation and haemorrhage source control should be performed, the latter with direct pressure over the area and use of tourniquets. The limb should be re-aligned which can also help to control the bleeding with repeat neurovascular assessment after this. Immediately escalate to the vascular surgery team if there are concerns about arterial injury. Consider CT angiogram. As per BOA standards, ischaemic limbs should be revascularized within four hours. If definitive arterial flow cannot be achieved, then an arterial shunt may be required. Based on the length of ischaemic time, intraoperative fasciotomies may be required. Postoperatively the patient should be assessed regularly for compartment syndrome [2].

How would you classify nerve injuries?

The Seddon classification is a way to assess peripheral nerve injury. It has three classes, in increasing severity and decreasing likelihood of complete return to premorbid function.

- Neuropraxia: temporary loss of conduction in a nerve without axonal discontinuity.
- Axonotmesis: loss of axon continuity but preserved connective tissue around it.
- Neurotmesis: loss of both the axon continuity and disrupted connective tissue architecture around it.

References

1. BOA (n.d.). 'BOAST – Open fractures'. Website, www.boa.ac.uk, www.boa.ac.uk/resource/boast-4-pdf.html.

2. BOA (n.d.). 'BOAST – Diagnosis & management of arterial injuries associated with extremity fractures and dislocations'. Website, www.boa.ac.uk, accessed 19 Feb. 2024, www.boa.ac.uk/resource/boast-6-pdf.html.

9.31 Painful Swollen Joint

You are the orthopaedic CT1 called to the emergency department to review an 11-year-old boy who has presented to the emergency department with a 1-day history of a painful hip, limiting his ability to walk. He is known to have T1DM. His hip is warm, red, and swollen. The child is tachycardic and febrile at 38.8°C, observations are otherwise stable. How do you proceed?

Before you begin: There are a range of paediatric hip conditions to be aware of, including developmental issues such as Perthe's disease, slipped upper femoral epiphysis (SUFE), and developmental dysplasia of the hip (DDH). Other differentials can be thought of as 'TTI', or 'tumour, trauma, infection'. The most concerning differential in this case considering a fever of 38.8°C is septic arthritis, particularly given the background of T1DM. This is an orthopaedic emergency which can result in irreversible articular cartilage damage and severe osteoarthritis. Mention this early in your answers. BOA standards are again available for this topic [1].

A–E

Airway
Breathing

- Give oxygen and ensure saturations are above 94% as part of the SEPSIS 6 protocol.

Circulation

- The patient is febrile and may also require operative management, so take full set of bloods including FBC (Kocher's criteria), U&Es, CRP (modified Kocher's criteria), ESR (Kocher's criteria), clotting, group and saves, blood cultures (ideally two sets), and VBG.
- Complete the SEPSIS 6 protocol (monitor urine output and give fluids as per paediatric guidelines). While antibiotics are typically given in SEPSIS 6 in cases of septic arthritis antibiotics may be held if the child is stable and surgery is planned, as deep tissue samples can be collected prior to commencing empiric treatment. However, as per BOA standards, children who meet high-risk sepsis criteria should have empiric IV abx started [1].

Disability

- Monitor sugars ± ketones which can derange in response to infection. If the patient is likely proceeding to theatre and will be made NBM for this, a VRII should be started.

Exposure

- Examination of the joint using a look/feel/move approach:
  - Look: acutely hot swollen tender joint, erythema. Hip held in flexion, abduction, and external rotation (this position maximises hip capsular volume)
  - Feel: temperature, effusion, crepitus.
  - Move: painful on both passive and active movement.

- Examination of patient's gait: inability to WB.
- Examination for possible causes of septic arthritis: full systematic examination, examination of spine, signs of endocarditis or recent trauma to the area.
- Always examine the joint above and below.

AAPS

- Stepwise approach to pain management, noting that decompressing the hip will ultimately help relieve the pain. Senior involvement in all cases of possible septic arthritis.

History, Notes, Investigation

- AMPLE history focusing on risk factors such as recent trauma to the area or joint procedures, as well as non-modifiable risk factors such as pre-existing joint disease, diabetes, immunosuppression, or chronic kidney disease.
- Ask about preceding history of viral illness (transient synovitis) or previous joint inflammation (juvenile polyarthritis).
- Bloods to calculate Kocher's criteria score (see below).
- Orthogonal view XRs of the affected joint – further imaging not typically needed in acute phase unless there is diagnostic uncertainty. Consider imaging joint above/below.

Preliminary Management

- Joint aspiration under aseptic technique with sample sent for urgent Gram stain and culture. Ultrasound is commonly used to guide hip aspirations.
- Following aspiration, commence empirical antibiotics as per local guidelines (note that these should be started immediately if the patient is septic/unstable).

Further Management

- Washout of joint (open or arthroscopic) in theatres is gold standard, and as per BOA standards should occur within 24 hours of diagnosis [1]. Debridement (e.g. synovectomy) may also be required.
- Antibiotics, typically intravenously for two weeks followed by four weeks oral, guided by sensitivities and discussion with microbiology.
- BOA standards also recommend that bone and joint injections should be followed up clinically and radiographically for a minimum of 12 months to aid identification of long-term complications [1].

Table 9.6 Kocher's criteria

Weight-bearing status	Non-weight-bearing status
Temperature	>38.5°C/101.3°F
ESR	>40 mm/hour
WBC	>12,000 cells/mm^3

N.B. the Modified Kocher's criteria is similar, but ESR is swapped for CRP (where a score of >20 mg/L is a positive score).

What complications arise with septic arthritis?
The infection can spread locally causing osteomyelitis, or systemically to cause sepsis. Damaged cartilage can cause osteoarthritis – pus is chondrolytic. Prolonged periods of infection and immobility can cause joint stiffness, chronic pain, a range of psychosocial issues, and VTE.

What organisms are commonly implicated in septic arthritis?
Most cases are caused by staphylococcal and streptococcal species, most commonly *Staphylococcus aureus*. In a sexually active patient gonococcal species should be considered. Puncture wounds or infections secondary to injected drug use are associated with *Pseudomonas*. *Salmonella* species are associated with patients with sickle cell disease.

What are Kocher's criteria?
A predictive tool used to help with the diagnosis of septic arthritis (Table 9.6). A score of 3 out of 4 constitutes a 93% chance of septic arthritis, all 4 gives a 99% chance of septic arthritis.

Reference

1. BOA (n.d.). 'BOAST – The management of children with acute musculoskeletal infection'. Website, www.boa.ac.uk, accessed 19 Feb. 2024, www.boa.ac.uk/ resource/boast-the-management-of-children-with-acute-musculoskeletal-infection.html#:~:text=Septic% 20arthritis%20requires%20surgical% 20drainage.

9.32 Post-tonsillectomy Bleeding

You are the ENT CT2 on call overnight and are bleeped by the ward to review a 15-year-old boy who is 4 hours post tonsillectomy and has started coughing up blood. How do you proceed?

Before you begin: You are being bleeped so remember to give instructions for the nursing staff over the phone; in this instance ask them to sit the patient up, take a set of observations, get the operation notes ready, and insert a cannula and take bloods if able. While the scenario is most likely a primary post-tonsillectomy bleed, you should start by mentioning other differentials you are concerned about, including upper GI bleed and pulmonary pathologies causing haemoptysis.

A–E
Airway
- The airway may be at risk; sit the patient up and lean them forward, ensuring they spit blood out into a sick bowl. If this is not possible, ensure they are turned onto their side to minimise the risk of them inhaling blood. Suctioning may be needed.
- Stress that any airway concerns would be escalated to anaesthetics and your registrar immediately.
- Remember to reassess the airway regularly, including after any interventions.

Breathing
- Ensure they are maintaining their saturations and have a normal RR, as they may already have inhaled a volume of blood.

Circulation
- Determine extent of bleeding and haemodynamic instability – escalate and proceed with major haemorrhage protocol if required. Examine the contents of the sick bowl to help assess the rate of bleeding.
- With a head torch and tongue depressor, examine the oral cavity and tonsillar fossa for active bleeding points or clots, estimating what proportion of the tonsillar fossa they cover. N.B. after a tonsillectomy, the tonsillar fossa usually is covered with a white-yellow pseuodomembrane which cannot be distinguished from post-tonsillectomy infection. A useful tip to see if there is active bleeding when the bleeding rate is very slow is to ask the patient to gargle with water and see what colour the water that they spit out is.
- In all cases, ensure the patient has wide bore IV access in each ACF and a full set of bloods, including FBC, VBG, clotting, and group and save has been sent.
- Begin preliminary management (see below).

Disability
Exposure
- Examine skin for signs of coagulopathy.

Extra Steps (AAPS)
- The registrar must be made aware of all cases of post-tonsillectomy bleeding.

History, Notes, Investigations
- History: full focused clinical history to assess bleeding history and postoperative course. In secondary bleeds, determining if the patient has been eating and drinking since the operation is key.
- Notes: assess previous documentation and operation notes (e.g. presence of recent or active infection during surgery, intraoperative issues with haemostasis and tonsillectomy technique used).

Preliminary Management

- Ice pack on the back of patient's neck.
- IV TXA: although this has no evidence in post-tonsillectomy bleeding, there is evidence it reduces the need for transfusion for surgical bleeding in general.
- H_2O_2 3% diluted in three parts water used to gargle: this can help to stop a slow bleed.
- Gauze and adrenaline: gauze swabs applied to the tonsillar fossa with a Magill forceps can help stem bleeding. Insert the gauze along the cheek and side of the mouth to avoid triggering the gag reflex and always keep the tail of the gauze outside the patient's mouth. It is useful to soak the gauze in 1:10,000 adrenaline solution for local vasoconstriction.
- Abx: as per local policy.
- Make the patient NBM.

Further Management

- Bleeding that is not quickly settling with simple measures necessitates operative management. Begin theatre workup (see Section 9.2).
- Even small bleeds should be admitted for observation for 24 hours. Close monitoring is needed as a small bleed may represent a herald bleed before a major haemorrhage.
- All patients should be reviewed by your registrar who will decide when the patient is safe for discharge, and when oral intake can be reintroduced.

What is the aetiology of post-tonsillectomy bleeding?
Primary bleeds (within the first 24 hours of the operation) usually relate to incomplete intraoperative haemostasis. Secondary bleeds (24 hours – 6 weeks postoperatively) usually relate to overlying infection, which occurs most commonly 4–10 days postoperatively. Eating solid food postoperatively is important to keep the tonsil bed clear of any debris, which may otherwise serve as a nidus for infection.

What may alert you to a post-tonsillectomy bleed in a young child?
In some instances a child may not present typically. There may be a history of blood found on their pillow, the parent may have noticed the child is swallowing excessively, or coughing up or vomiting blood.

What intraoperative measures can be used to prevent primary post-tonsillectomy bleeding?
Meticulous haemostasis should be performed intraoperatively. Particular attention should be given to the main vascular pedicle situated on the inferior pole of the tonsil, which may need hand tying. The tonsil (Boyle–Davis) gag can be loosened after the tonsillectomy and the area re-checked after a short pause to ensure no bleeding has started after the tissues have been relaxed.

9.33 Painful Groin Lump

You are called to assess a 65-year-old obese man in the emergency department who presents with constant severe pain in his right groin for the last three hours with an associated tender lump. He looks generally well but is complaining of agonising pain. Aside from elevated HR (116 bpm) his observations are normal. How do you proceed?

Before you begin: Groin lumps have a wide differential, but the timeframe, the patient being an older male, and the constant pain seemingly out of proportion to the clinical picture should make you concerned for a strangulated hernia. Other differentials can be thought of via an anatomical layers approach: skin (epidermoid cysts, skin cancers), subcutaneous (lipoma, lymph nodes), muscle (sarcoma), vascular (saphena varix, aortic, iliac or femoral artery aneurysm), and urological (undescended testicle which is torting). Candidates should be confident on types of hernia and basic inguinal anatomy in case of a follow-up question on this – in the interest of space, this book does not cover anatomy.

A–E
Airway
Breathing
Circulation
- Fluid resuscitation as required.
- Wide bore IV access in each ACF and full set of bloods including FBC, U&E, CRP, VBG (note the lactate here is crucial), group and saves, and clotting for potential theatre preparation.
- ECG for tachycardia.
- Catheterise to monitor fluid output.

Disability
- Temperature – strangulation is classically associated with fever.

Exposure
- Full abdominal examination, including a PR exam. A full lump exam should be performed, in this instance looking for signs that the hernia is incarcerated (tense, tender, irreducible) or strangulated (as before but peritonitic, pain out of proportion to clinical signs). An inguinal hernia will be superomedial to the pubic tubercle. A femoral hernia will be inferolateral to the pubic tubercle.

AAPS
- 'Agonising pain' is mentioned, so suitable analgesia must be given – IV morphine may be appropriate in the first instance if this can be given. This may be contributing to his tachycardia. Your senior will need to be aware of this patient urgently.

History, Notes, Investigations
- AMPLE history, with focus on hernia risk factors (obesity, causes of increased intra-abdominal pressure such as constipation, coughing, and heavy lifting) and bowel obstruction symptoms.
- Radiology including US or CT abdomen-pelvis with contrast (which can help exclude other differentials).

Preliminary Management

- Attempt to reduce the hernia with analgesia and patient in the Trendelenburg position. If this is not successful, a strangulated hernia will need to proceed to operative management, so make the patient NBM and begin operative workup (see Section 9.2).
- If the patient is also in small bowel obstruction then commence drip and suck.

Further Management

- Urgent surgical exploration, reduction of the hernia, and repair of the hernial defect. The type of repair used varies based on the size and anatomy of the hernia, the level of contamination and the surgeon's personal preference. While mesh can decrease the rate of postoperative recurrence, using this in the context of strangulation with necrosis or enteric contamination increases the risk of postoperative infection.

What is the difference between an indirect and direct inguinal hernia?
Both represent the protrusion of abdominal viscera through the anterior abdominal wall into the inguinal canal. Indirect hernias (80%) occur due to a failure of the processus vaginalis to close; bowel enters the inguinal cavity via the deep inguinal ring, lateral to the inferior epigastric vessels. Direct hernias (20%) occur when bowel herniates directly through a weakness in the abdominal wall, medial to the inferior epigastric vessels, in Hesselbach's triangle. Indirect hernias tend to occur in paediatric patients, direct hernias in older patients. They can be reliably differentiated intraoperatively by observing their relationship to the inferior epigastric vessels.

What postoperative complications would you consent the patient for?
If I felt competent to consent the patient, I would warn them about general operative risks, such as the risks of bleeding, infection, haematoma, VTE, and the risks of a general anaesthetic. Specific complications would include the risks of recurrence, chronic groin pain lasting greater than three months, damage to nearby structures such as the vas deferens or testicular vessels, subfertility, paraesthesia, and mesh migration/erosion.

How would the scenario differ if you were reviewing a stable patient in an outpatient clinic with a reducible inguinal hernia?
I would still ensure the patient was stable with an A–E workup. If I was uncertain about the diagnosis, I would ensure my senior had reviewed; an ultrasound may be ordered as a diagnostic adjunct. I would counsel the patient on the management options. If the patient is minimally symptomatic, conservative management may be appropriate. However, I would counsel them on a strangulation risk of around 2% per year and explain the signs of incarceration and strangulation to look out for. If the patient proceeds to an elective repair, this may be using an open approach with mesh or suture repair. If the hernia is bilateral or recurrent a laparoscopic approach is typically used, although primary unilateral hernias may be managed laparoscopically in the first instance in patients deemed higher risk of developing chronic pain.

How would management of the scenario differ if you were reviewing a stable one-year-old baby in an outpatient clinic with a soft umbilical hernia?

I would ensure the child was stable from an A–E workup. If I was confident with the diagnosis of an umbilical hernia, I would explain to the parents that this is a common condition affecting 30% of babies, associated with certain risk factors such as prematurity and low birthweight, which tend to close spontaneously within three years. I would counsel them on the signs of incarceration, strangulation, and bowel obstruction. If there are concerns beyond this point, we usually consider operative repair around four or five years of age.

What other abdominal hernias do you know about?

- Femoral: inferolateral to pubic tubercle, high chance of obstruction/strangulation, therefore ideally repaired operatively within two weeks.
- Epigastric: midline from xiphoid to umbilicus, usually only contain preperitoneal fat.
- Spigelian: rare protrusion of abdominal contents through Spigelian fascia (formed of the transversus abdominus and internal oblique aponeuroses).
- Obturator: rare herniation through obturator canal situated on the anterolateral wall of the pelvis.
- Incisional: herniation through sites of previous surgical access to abdominal cavity.
- Hiatus: herniation through a defect in the diaphragm into the thoracic cavity.

9.34 Postoperative Fall in Urine Output

You are the general surgical CT1 covering the wards. A 78-year-old man is on day 5 after a partial hepatectomy. The nurse calls you to report he has not passed urine into his catheter bag in the past eight hours. His observations are unremarkable. How would you approach this patient?

Before you begin: Ask the nurse to ensure his notes and fluid balance chart are at the bedside, that a new set of observations are taken, and that the patient has IV access. You can consider the causes of a fall in urine output through the lens of pre-renal, renal, and post-renal causes.

A–E
Airway
Breathing
Circulation

- Ensure the patient has adequate IV access with wide bore cannulae and start a bag of IV crystalloid fluid.
- A full set of bloods should be taken, including a VBG and U&Es to check eGFR.
- Assess their fluid balance, including reviewing their fluid chart.
- Look for signs of haemorrhage postoperatively including by inspecting abdominal drains and also signs of sepsis (chest, abdomen, wound site, lines, catheter-associated UTI particularly).

- Check the catheter to ensure it is draining, including by flushing the catheter and aspirating, and feeling for a palpable bladder.

Disability
Exposure

AAPS

History, Notes, Investigation
- Take a thorough history from the patient about fluid intake, known renal impairment, symptoms of systemic infection, and review notes to check for pre-existing renal disease.
- Review and hold medications that may cause acute tubular necrosis or are nephrotoxic.
- Urine dip.
- Bladder scan.

Preliminary Management
- If the patient has become suddenly anuric, the most likely issue is a blocked catheter. This is supported by a bladder scan showing a raised volume in the bladder. This should be flushed or reinserted to unblock it. Once draining, urine should be inspected for signs of infection or clots.
- If this fails to resolve the anuria, then all nephrotoxic medications should be held.
- If the patient is clinically dry, then address the underlying cause, provide replacement fluids and monitor for a response to the fluids. A strict input/output monitoring chart should be kept.

What is your differential for postoperative drop in urine output?
- Pre-renal: Hypovolaemia, haemorrhage, sepsis. Note that patients often have a drop in urine output after operations due to blood loss, and a physiological stress response which includes the activation of the renin-angiotensin-aldosterone axis, and also release of ADH. This typically should not last more than 24 hours.
- Renal: Acute glomerulonephritis, acute tubular necrosis (including nephrotoxicity due to medications), acute tubulo-interstitial nephritis.
- Post-renal: Blocked catheter, bladder outlet obstruction (particularly in un-catheterised elderly male patients), acute urinary retention or acute on chronic urinary retention.

How might you differentiate pre-renal and intrinsic renal causes?
This would be done with a mixture of a thorough history as detailed above, as well as examination findings, bedside observations/investigations, and response to a fluid challenge. In a prerenal AKI you would expect signs of hypovolaemia, and an appropriate increase in urine output in response to a fluid challenge. In an intrinsic renal AKI you often see normal or elevated BP, normal volume status, no effect from a fluid challenge and findings such as blood/protein on a urine dip and pathology-specific findings on a urine microscopy. In neither case should you find a full bladder on bladder scanning.

At what urine output would you consider the patient to be oliguric?
Less than 0.5 ml/kg/hour of urine output for six hours is oliguria as per the RIFLE criteria.

What are the risk factors for postoperative oliguria?
- Preoperative factors: age, chronic kidney disease or known renal dysfunction, ischaemic heart disease or heart failure, and diabetes.
- Intraoperative factors: emergency surgery, prolonged surgery, intraperitoneal or intrathoracic surgery, need for red blood cell transfusion, usage of inotropes, operation-specific factors such as aortic cross clamp time in an AAA repair.
- Postoperative: use of nephrotoxic drugs, diuretic use, inadequate fluid intake.

What are some indications for urgent renal replacement therapy?
- Resistant hyperkalaemia.
- Resistant acid-base disturbance (metabolic acidosis).
- Refractory pulmonary oedema/fluid overload.
- Severe symptomatic uraemia causing encephalopathy or pericarditis.

9.35 Hip Dislocation

You are the orthopaedic CT1 on call and are asked to assess a 21-year-old male who was the driver in a head-on road traffic accident. He is complaining of groin pain as well as numbness in his leg on the right side, and an inability to weight bear. His leg is internally rotated and adducted. He is otherwise stable. How would you approach the management of this patient?

Before you begin: This case history is concerning for a 'dashboard injury' in which the axial load through a flexed and adducted hip can cause a posterior hip dislocation. This can damage the sciatic nerve. Posterior dislocations require considerable force in the native hip of a young patient; ensure a trauma call has been put out and look for other injuries such as ipsilateral injuries to the femoral head, femoral neck, and acetabulum. You should rattle off a comprehensive and precise ATLS A–E to rule out these concomitant injuries.

A–E
C-Spine
Airway
Breathing
Circulation
Disability
Exposure
- Full top-to-toe examination including log roll to identify concomitant injuries, followed by a look, feel, move approach to examination of the hip.
- Look for arthroplasty scars (previous arthroplasty is a key risk factor for hip dislocation), obvious bony deformity, bruising/skin changes, and breaches of skin integrity. Posterior hip dislocation generally produces an internally rotated and adducted hip. Feel for tenderness, haematomas/collections, and examine the downstream pulses (dorsalis pedis

and posterior tibial) and neurology (particularly the sciatic nerve, which is impinged in 10%–20% cases; examine for the function of the tibial, superficial peroneal, and deep peroneal branches). Examine the active and passive ranges of motion – but be wary of the pain this may cause the patient. Always examine the joint above (sacroiliac/lower back) and below (knee).

AAPS
– Ensure adequate analgesia, particularly if considering attempting reduction.

History, Notes, Investigation
– AMPLE history including details about the mechanism of injury.
– Given the high energy required to cause posterior hip dislocation, a trauma CT may be warranted. A CT will also help rule out concurrent fractures, and help guide reduction. Otherwise, orthogonal view XRs will be needed.

Preliminary and Further Management
– Closed reduction of dislocation in the first instance. Note that you are not expected to be competent to reduce and manage this alone, but you should know to call for senior support, as well as the general principles of dislocation management. Post reduction XR is used to confirm relocation.
– A CT scan should be requested for all native hip dislocation, following reduction, to assess for loose bodies, as well as allowing assessment of concomitant injuries.
– Patients with isolated hip dislocation typically have protected weight bearing for four to six weeks.

What are the general steps in managing a dislocated joint?
– Examine the joint, document neurovascular status before and after you do anything, obtain imaging as required.
– Attempt to relocate the joint with traction and counter-traction.
– Reassess neurovascular status and repeat imaging.
– If reduced – consider mobilisation plan and follow-up requirements.
– If not reduced – consider manipulation under anaesthesia or open reduction in theatre.

What is the difference between dislocation and subluxation?
Both refer to abnormal separation of a joint. In subluxation, some contact between articular surfaces remains. In dislocation, no contact remains.

What are some common associated injuries with a posterior hip dislocation?
Sciatic nerve injury, femoral head, femoral neck, and acetabular fractures, ipsilateral lower limb injuries.

How would you read the radiograph and what are the XR findings for a posteriorly dislocated hip?
I would confirm demographic details to ensure the correct patient, date, and side. I would ensure there were orthogonal views of the hip (AP and lateral). I would confirm the

radiograph spanned from above the iliac crest to one third down the femoral shaft. I would then inspect the bones looking at the cortical outline, bony texture and looking for asymmetry to reveal any fractures or joint disruption. I would inspect the elements of the femur, the pelvis and their relative positions. I would trace Shenton's line and the three pelvic rings for discontinuity. I would assess the joints to ensure the correct relation of the articulating bones and appropriate joint spaces. I would do this for the acetabular, pubic symphysis, and sacroiliac joints. Finally, I would assess the soft tissues. In this case, I would expect to find disruption of Shenton's line and loss of congruence between femoral head and acetabulum. The posteriorly dislocated hip will look smaller and superimpose on the roof of the acetabulum. Internal rotation will reduce the visualisation of the femur.

What complications are associated with posterior hip dislocations?
Immediate complications include neurovascular damage – namely sciatic nerve injury which would cause foot drop and altered lower limb sensation. Later complications include avascular necrosis of the femoral head (particularly if reduction is delayed), post-traumatic arthritis (up to 20%), and recurrent dislocations (<2%).

9.36 Painful Calf

You are the orthopaedic CT1 called to the inpatient ward to review an 80-year-old female patient who had a left hemiarthroplasty for a fractured neck of femur. She is now post-operative day 4. She has remained in bed since the operation, her patient-controlled analgesia was stopped yesterday, she refuses to wear stockings or receive any injections. She is now complaining of a painful left leg, particularly in the calf. How would you approach this patient?

Before you begin: This history is concerning for a DVT. The differential also includes an acutely ischaemic limb, cellulitis, and a missed fracture of the lower limb. Stress the urgency of the situation and review them immediately. You should be mentioning the Wells' criteria.

A–E
Airway
Breathing
- Assess RR, O_2 sats and for respiratory distress to concurrently assess for a pulmonary embolus.

Circulation
- Ensure wide bore IV access obtained.
- Full set of bloods, including clotting and D-dimer.
- ECG (in case of PE or arrythmia).

Disability
Exposure
- Examination of the affected area with a look, feel, move approach, looking for key signs of a DVT. Reference that you are assessing the leg as per the Well's criteria:

measure calf size with a tape measure, check for entire leg swelling, collateral non-varicose veins, localised tenderness along the deep venous system, and pitting oedema, confined to the leg in question.
– Document neurovascular status, and particularly distal pulses.

AAPS
– Analgesia as per WHO pain ladder being wary of renal and hepatic function in this elderly patient. The operating surgeon (or your registrar) should be made aware of postoperative VTE events.

History, Notes, Investigation
Take a full AMPLE history before focusing on the other elements of Well's criteria such as previous confirmed VTE or active cancer, as well as assessing for respiratory symptoms that may point to a VTE. The history will also help to exclude other differentials.

What are risk factors for VTE?
Risk factors for VTE can be split into Virchow's triad of endothelial dysfunction (e.g. vascular damage intraoperatively), venous stasis (postoperative immobility, prior venous disease), and coagulopathy (postoperative inflammatory states, prior history of coagulopathy).

Is a D-dimer useful in this situation?
A D-dimer is usually taken as part of the workup for possible VTEs. It is a low specificity test, and many other things can elevate it, including infection, inflammation, liver disease, and pregnancy. In the perioperative period, a D-dimer is less useful given it will be raised following recent surgery or trauma.

Preliminary and Further Management of DVT (NICE Guidelines [1])
I would conduct a two-level Wells score in this patient. If they scored greater than or equal to two, I would consider a DVT likely and aim for a proximal lower limb ultrasound to be performed within four hours. If this was not possible I would take a D-dimer, then give interim therapeutic anticoagulation while waiting for the ultrasound, which should be performed within 24 hours. If the patient's Wells score was less than 2, a DVT would be unlikely, and I would perform a D-dimer only. If this was positive, I would give interim therapeutic anticoagulation and request an urgent proximal ultra-sound of the limb.

If a clot were confirmed, I would consult local guidelines on anticoagulation pathways, but likely I would offer rivaroxaban or apixaban first line. Prior to prescribing, I would discuss this with a senior, noting that if the patient was at high risk of bleeding, then a reversible agent such as heparin may be more suitable. I would request baseline blood tests including full blood count, renal and hepatic function, prothrombin time (PT), and APTT. I would then organise three-month follow-up in anticoagulation clinic.

I would safety-net the patient and advise them when to seek medical attention in future. I would ensure the patient was suitably counselled on how to use anticoagulants, about the duration of treatment, possible adverse effects, and interactions associated with anticoagulation treatment. I would tell the patient how anticoagulants may affect their dental treatment, about the risks associated with extended travel and the need to avoid high-risk activities.

What are the components of the Wells' criteria?

You would be unlikely to be asked to list off the full Wells' criteria in an interview. However, it's a useful scoring system to know, and any candidate who can weave some of its components into their assessment will stand out.

– Risk factors: active cancer, bedridden >3 days or major surgery within 12 weeks, paralysis, or recent leg immobilisation, previous DVT.
– Examination: calf swelling >3 cm vs other leg, collateral superficial veins present (non-varicose), entire leg swollen, localised tenderness along deep venous system, pitting oedema in symptomatic leg only.
– Other diagnosis as or more likely than DVT deducts two points.

Reference

1. National Institute for Health and Care Excellence (2020). 'Overview | Venous thromboembolic diseases: Diagnosis, management and thrombophilia testing | Guidance | NICE'. Website, www.nice.org.uk, www.nice.org.uk/guidance/ng158.

9.37 Flank Pain

You are the on-call Urology CT1 and are called to see a 78-year-old man in A&E. He presented with acute onset severe right-sided colicky abdominal pain. He is known to have previously suffered from a ureteric stone. HR 110, BP 110/70, pyrexial (38.7°C), RR 18, 98% on room air. What is your differential in this case and how would you proceed?

Before you begin: This history is worrying for an infected obstructed stone. However, do not forget that a ruptured abdominal aortic aneurysm is another 'must not miss' differential in this case.

Differential

This patient sounds acutely unwell, and I would review them immediately, taking a CCRISP A–E approach. My top differential would include an infected obstructed urinary system secondary to a ureteric stone. The other most important differential to consider is a ruptured abdominal aortic aneurysm. Both are life-threatening emergencies. I would categorise other differentials by system. Urinary causes include pyelonephritis, lower urinary tract infection, renal abscess, renal artery aneurysm. GI causes include diverticulitis, mesenteric ischaemia, pancreatitis, small bowel obstruction. Vascular causes include symptomatic abdominal aortic aneurysm and mycotic aneurysms.

A–E

Airway
Breathing

– Commence SEPSIS 6 management by starting patient on high-flow O_2.

Circulation

- Wide bore IV access, bloods including VBG, FBC, U&Es, clotting, group and saves, and blood cultures.
- Commence fluids resuscitation titrated to response.
- Catheterise and send urine MC&S.

Disability
Exposure

- Focused abdominal examination, in particular checking for: renal angle tenderness, loin to groin pain, palpable bladder. Assess for signs of a AAA.

AAPS

- PR Diclofenac is the preferred analgesia method for renal colic pain. Remember that in a younger female patient a pregnancy test is essential with this history to exclude an ectopic pregnancy.

History, Notes, Investigation

- AMPLE history focusing on characterising the pain (colicky pain in stones vs dull pain of pyelonephritis), preceding lower urinary tract symptoms, and risk factors, previous history, and family history, of urinary stone disease.
- A CTKUB looking for signs of an infected obstructed system, such as: hydronephrosis and perinephric or periureteric fat stranding.

The CT scan confirms an obstructing stone with signs of infection. What is your definitive management of this patient?

An infected obstructed system is a urological emergency. In addition to commencing SEPSIS 6, a decision should be made about how the urinary tract will be decompressed, either with nephrostomy or with ureteric stenting. The decision should be made by discussing with the urology registrar on call; while evidence suggests no difference in outcomes between these options, local availability and patient-specific contraindications for each approach should be considered. I would prepare the patient for CEPOD. Intraoperatively, a sample of urine should be sent from the infected system.

After the system has been decompressed, ureteroscopy is typically performed four to six weeks later to clear the obstructing stone, after which the stent/nephrostomy can be removed. Depending on the subsequent stone analysis, I would ensure the patient were reviewed in clinic to provide lifestyle advice or treatment to reduce the high risk of recurrence of stone formation.

What compositions of ureteric stone are you aware of?

- Calcium stones including calcium oxalate, calcium phosphate.
- Uric acid stones.
- Struvite stones.
- Cysteine stones.
- Rarer compositions include xanthine stones (genetic), drug-induced stones (e.g. antiretrovirals in HIV such as indinavir), and matrix stones (organic materials associated with UTI).

What are some modifiable risk factors for stone formation?

This depends on the type of stone. Common risk factors include dehydration, poor oral intake, high protein intake, high oxalate intake (berries, chocolate, spinach, beans), and high salt intake. Futhermore, urinary tract infections can increase the risk of struvite stones, while alcohol comsumption can increase the risk of uric acid stones.

Note: the question specifically asks for modifiable risk factors, therefore do not list age/sex/family history!

Chapter 1

Concluding Remarks

By going through these cases we hope that you have developed:

- A consistent structured A–E approach for both acute and trauma cases, which you can tailor to the specific case at hand.
- Mini-scripts for common sub-scenarios, such as resuscitation of a septic patient, examination of a limb, or working a patient up for CEPOD, which you can comfortably fall back on when required.
- A structured approach to answering follow-up questions.
- Confidence in handling variations in interviewer technique, such as being interrupted mid-case, or being moved on quickly to a latter part of the case.

The scenarios presented have covered a diverse range of topics, but naturally it is impossible to predict all the scenarios that might come up. However, whatever stations do come up, it is almost certain you will need to be able to perform a comprehensive A–E assessment, and this should always remain your focus when preparing for the clinical stations. We hope that the tools and frameworks you have gained from the textbook will help you tackle any case that comes up, even those you have not previously practised. Be confident, be engaging and above all, be prepared. We wish you the best of luck.

Index